ORAL HEALTH SEEKING BEHAVIOR

SHRUDHA POTDAR
SIDDANA GOUD R
NAGESH L

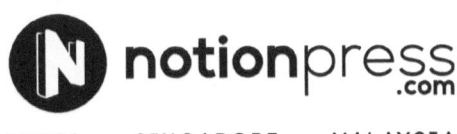

INDIA • SINGAPORE • MALAYSIA

Notion Press

Old No. 38, New No. 6
McNichols Road, Chetpet
Chennai - 600 031

First Published by Notion Press 2019
Copyright © Shrudha Potdar, Siddana Goud R, Nagesh L 2019
All Rights Reserved.

ISBN 978-1-64587-547-5

This book has been published with all efforts taken to make the material error-free after the consent of the authors. However, the authors and the publisher do not assume and hereby disclaim any liability to any party for any loss, damage, or disruption caused by errors or omissions, whether such errors or omissions result from negligence, accident, or any other cause.

While every effort has been made to avoid any mistake or omission, this publication is being sold on the condition and understanding that neither the authors nor the publishers or printers would be liable in any manner to any person by reason of any mistake or omission in this publication or for any action taken or omitted to be taken or advice rendered or accepted on the basis of this work. For any defect in printing or binding the publishers will be liable only to replace the defective copy by another copy of this work then available.

CONTENTS

Why Oral Health Seeking Behavior imperative?..5

Definitions..9

1. Health Seeking Behavior Models...13
2. Oral Health Seeking Behavior Models 29
3. Critiques of Health Seeking Behavior Models 35
4. Barriers Affecting Oral Health Seeking Behavior 37
5. Overcoming Barriers to Oral Health Seeking Behavior 46
6. Factors Affecting Health Seeking Behavior 62

Summary & Take Away Notes 95

References 97

WHY ORAL HEALTH SEEKING BEHAVIOR IMPERATIVE?

In the words of Nobel laureate Amartya Sen, Health, like Education is among the basic capabilities which give value to human life.

Health is just not merely the lack of disease; the concept of health goes beyond the absence of disease and comprises of physical, psychological, behavioral and social components which follows a holistic concept. It also contributes to the social and economic prosperity; therefore it is important to protect health through health care. Health in itself has a great value as it enables people to enjoy their potential as human beings. The link between health and human behavior is a major area of interest in public health. Human behavior frequently influences the Health seeking behavior of individuals. Health seeking behavior is described as the activities undertaken by an individual in response to disease symptoms experienced. It also describes all those things an individual does to prevent and detect diseases in asymptomatic stages in order to find an appropriate remedy.[1] Understanding Health seeking behavior is very difficult and complex to ascertain and establish.

Oral health forms an integral component of general health because both 'Health' as well as 'Oral health' are related to the functional, psychological, social and aesthetic well-being of a person. Consequently oral health seeking behavior could be considered as a part of general health seeking behavior. Oral health problems affect all age groups and are universal in prevalence. Utilization of dental services, availability of dental services, accessibility to oral health as well as affordability determines the oral health seeking behavior of individuals. Regular utilisation of dental services has been considered to be an important health behavior which means seeking preventive dental care well before symptoms appear.[2] The availability and accessibility of oral health services are seriously inhibited and the provision of essential oral care is limited in many developing countries including India. Very low utilization of oral health care services and less number of visits to a dental-care facility are probably due to lack of confidence in oral health professionals which make people hesitant to seek professional help. Globalization, political instability, poverty and unemployment in economically deprived areas are some of the important factors that contribute to this phenomenon.

Social disparities in health and oral health outcomes as measured by education, occupation, income and household assets or by indices derived by combining indicators constitute one of the main challenges for Public health. People living in the rural areas are deprived of oral health services due to low geographical access. Ethnic beliefs and values may act to reinforce or inhibit the use of health services, depending upon their perceptions towards health.[3] Lower socio-economic and ethnic minority groups are less likely to utilize health services. Dental utilization patterns of older adults of minority groups are very less as compared to elders of other groups. There is increasing demand for care among people of all age groups and there is limited availability of resources. Increased emphasis on oral health promotion and disease prevention appears to be the only feasible response. Access to a usual source of dental care is influenced by both delivery system characteristics and personal resources. Equality in health care services means similar right to use services regardless of social status, economic resources or place of residence.[4] Equal utilization for equal need has been accepted more generally as a goal and therefore the principle of equity has to be introduced. In spite of the available health facilities in communities, there is still poor utilization of dental services due to various reasons.[5] Hence, there is an urgent need to know about the health related behaviors. More emphasis should be laid on the utility of dental services and behavioral antecedents of oral health seeking behaviors such as predisposing, enabling and reinforcing factors in behavior change communication. Thus, an attempt is made in this Book to know all the aspects of oral health seeking behavior, and to have a thorough knowledge of oral health seeking behavior through systematic literature search.

DEFINITIONS

1. Health

Health is the state of complete physical, mental and social well-being and not merely the absence of disease or infirmity, the ability to lead a "socially and economically productive life". (WHO, 1978).

Health is said to refer to a state of well-being or a restorative situation that is culturally constituted, defined, valued, and practiced by individuals or groups that enables them to function in their daily lives. (Leininger and McFarland, 2002).

2. Illness

Illness is an unhealthy condition or an abnormal process in which aspects of the social, physical, emotional, or intellectual condition and function of a person are diminished or impaired compared with that of the person's previous condition. (Mosby's Medical Dictionary, 2009).

Illness is defined in almost the same way as a disease or indisposition or a state of ill health. (The Collins English Dictionary, 2006).

3. Behavior

Behavior is deportment or conduct; any or all of a person's total activity especially that which is externally observable. (Dorland's Medical Dictionary for Health Consumers, 2007). Behavior is defined as all of the activities of a person, including physical actions which are observed directly and mental activities which are inferred and interpreted. (Mosby's Medical Dictionary, 2009).

4. Health seeking behavior

Health seeking behaviors are personal actions to promote optimal wellness, recovery, and rehabilitation. (Mosby's Medical Dictionary 2009).

Health seeking behaviors are the activities undertaken by individuals in response to disease symptoms experienced. (Collins English Dictionary 2006).

5. Care

A process of providing to people what they need for their health or protection. (The Oxford Dictionary, 2000).

6. Self-care

Self-care is the personal and medical care performed by the patient, usually in collaboration with and after instruction by a health care professional. (Mosby's Medical Dictionary, 2009).

7. Barriers (synonym: obstacle)

Any condition that makes it difficult to make progress or to achieve an objective.

8. Informal health care

Informal health care is the care sought from other channels of health care delivery systems such as traditional healers apart from formal health care facilities where the health care is given by health care professionals or other trained health professionals such as community health workers.

9. Self-care health seeking behavior

Self-care health seeking behaviors is treatment prescribed by self or rather self-medication. Informal care given by significant others in the family to siblings or other members of the family also falls under self-care health seeking behaviors. Included also in this group is the care sought from the informal sector, for instance, pharmacists, drug vendors and traditional healers such as divine healers, herbalists and witchdoctors.

10. Dental services

Multitude of services provided to individuals or communities by agents of health service or professions for the purpose of promotion, maintaining, monitoring or restoring health.

11. Dental care utilization

Dental care utilization is the percentage of the population who access dental services over a specified period. (Brown LJ, 1999).

12. Utilization

It is the actual attendance by members of the public at dental treatment facilities to receive dental care. Utilization is expressed as the proportion of a population who attended a dentist within a given time, usually a year, or as the average number of visits per person made during a year.

HEALTH SEEKING BEHAVIOR MODELS

A Brief Overview

A variety of factors impact health behavior and ultimately the health status. Education, cultural awareness, social support programs and public policies can have great impact on the evolution of attitudes, perceptions, knowledge and practices that improve oral health. Models have been proposed to assist in understanding the factors associated with general and oral health behavior, clinical status and satisfaction of individuals about health. Health and treatment-seeking behavior models from social psychology, medical sociology and medical anthropology are utilized in behavioral studies related to knowledge, attitude and practices.

In public health, probably the most utilized models from social psychology include the Health Belief Model followed by the Theory of Reasoned Action and its later development to the Theory of Planned Behavior. Most known health seeking behavior models from medical sociology and medical anthropology are, respectively, the Health Care Utilization or Socio-Behavioral Model by Andersen and the Decision Making Models. All models contain associations of variables which are considered relevant for explaining or predicting health-seeking behaviors. Few health seeking behavior models are considered in research designs to serve as a catalogue to understand behavior of individuals.

The main statistical data obtained using these models permit the evaluation of the relative weight of different factors in health behavior (use of preventive or therapeutic measures, choice between different health resources, non-compliance with treatment, or the consequences of behavior for delayed care seeking). The principal objective is to identify problematic areas in order to intervene with specific health system strategies. Very frequently, investigators adapt the models to the peculiarities of their research field or study area, or fuse various models, with the main aim to increase the range of possible key factors rather than to achieve theoretical advancements. Various models have been proposed to understand health seeking behavior which are listed below as follows:

I. The Health Belief Model (HBM)

II. The Theory of Reasoned action

III. The Theory of Planned Behavior

IV. The Health care utilization model

V. Variant of Health care utilization model (Kroegers et al)

VI. The Four A's Model

VII. Pathway Model

VIII. Social Cognition Model

IX. Conceptual Framework (Modified from Anderson)

I. The Health Belief Model (HBM)

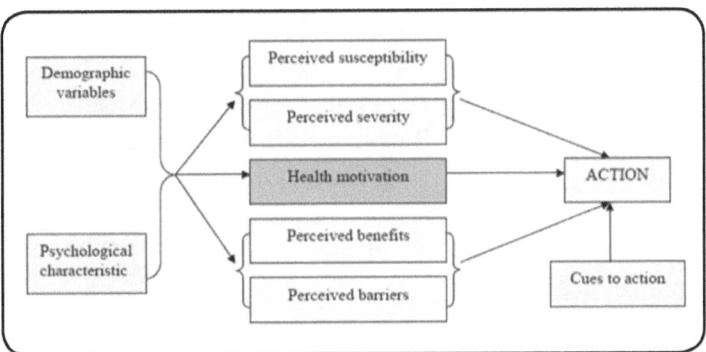

FIGURE 1

Figure 1 shows the HBM presented by **Sheeran and Abraham (1995)**.[6] **Health** Belief Model (HBM) was one of the first attempts to view health within a social context. The underlying principle of the HBM is that individuals with better information make better health decisions. According to **Hockbaum,** people will find it worthwhile when making health related decisions to keep an open mind. A person who is prepared to accept new concepts, will have a better understanding of self. With a better understanding of how and why they make choices, individuals will be much better able to make them intelligently, independently and maturely. The HBM is a staged theory, with each step in the decision making process dependent on the previous decision or belief. According to this theory, an individual must believe that she/he is susceptible to a condition; the condition is serious; there is a successful intervention for the condition; and can overcome all barriers to using the intervention. Each step is dependent on the previous belief. Applying this theory to an oral health condition such as early childhood caries, the primary caregiver must believe that the child is susceptible to dental caries; that primary teeth are important and dental caries is a serious threat to them; that dental caries can be prevented; and must be willing to limit the child's exposure to fermentable carbohydrates, and must assist the child in practicing good oral hygiene.

According to **Sheeran and Abraham** action in the HBM is guided by[6]:

1. Beliefs about the impact of illness and its consequences (threat perception) which depend on:

    Perceived susceptibility, or the beliefs about how vulnerable a person considers himself or herself in relation to a certain illness or health problem.

    Perceived severity of illness or health problems and its consequences;

2. **Health motivation,** or readiness to be concerned about health matters.

3. Beliefs about the consequences of health practices and about the possibilities and the effort to put them into practice. The behavioral evaluation depends on:

    Perceived benefits of preventive or therapeutic health practices;

    Perceived barriers, both material and psychological (for example 'will-power'), with regard to a certain health practice.

4. **Cues to action**, which includes different, internal and external factors, which influence action. For example, the nature and intensity (organic and symbolic) of illness symptoms, mass media campaigns, advice from relevant others. (family, friends, health staff and so on).

5. Beliefs and health motivation are conditioned by **socio-demographic variables** (class, age, gender, religion, etc.) and by the **psychological characteristics** of the interviewed person (personality, peer group pressure and so on).

A **limitation** of the HBM is that supplying information alone is usually not enough to change health behaviors. Behavior changes rarely follow a logical, stepwise progression. Cross sectional studies have found strong associations between good oral health and HBM stages. However, longitudinal studies have not shown good predictive value in following HBM principles. It is possible that measuring health beliefs cross sectionally reveals that, after a behavior is adopted, the individual believes the condition is serious and that interventions have value. However, measuring those beliefs before behavior changes take place has questionable value. Health belief model is possibly the most known model in public health, and also the oldest one from social psychology.

II. The Theory of Reasoned Action

Theory of Reasoned Action stresses the importance of attitudes and intentions in changing a behavior. According to this theory, the most important determinant of behavior is intention. Very few actions that produce a healthy outcome happen without sufficient knowledge and full intention to practice the healthy behavior.

Two cognitive processes are at work to develop healthy behaviors:

a. Belief about what significant others think.

b. Personal motivation to comply with those significant people.

Other external variables that will influence attitudes and thus behaviors are internally processed within the context of significance. According to the Theory of Reasoned Action, people make rational decisions based on their knowledge, personal values and attitudes. Therefore, a person's intent to perform a certain action is the most immediate and relevant predictor of carrying out that action. **Behavioral beliefs** and **normative beliefs** are two kinds of beliefs that shape intentions.[6]

a. **Behavioral beliefs** are the attitudes held by the individual alone. A person forms attitudes based on relative risks, benefits and possible outcomes. Therefore, personal knowledge and perception of personal health importance influence behavioral beliefs.

b. **Normative beliefs** are those held by other people who influence the individual. If a certain behavior is expected or is the social norm, or is expected by someone of importance to the individual, those expectations will have a bearing on an individual's intentions and, therefore, affect his or her behavior.

Limitations of this theory:

1. Intentions will only predict behavior if they are stable and consistent. When faced with an unexpected obstacle, an individual might change his or her intentions and neglect to carry out the originally intended behavior.

2. Intentions must be matched very closely to the behavior to have predictive power.

Social norms and community expectations are powerful predictors of individual behavior, according to the Theory of Reasoned Action. When using this theory in a community intervention, the behavior of the collective community may be more easily predicted than that of the individual. Social norms do not change as readily as individual choices; therefore, social norms are more stable and provide strong normative beliefs to those in a close community. The Theory of Reasoned Action helps explain an individual's perceptions of normal and expected behavior. The theory seems to be most successful in predicting behaviors that are completely within the individual's control and in which intentions remain stable, such as daily oral hygiene practices. Extraneous factors outside of the individual's control, such as fatigue or change of environment, may quickly change intentions and therefore change behavior and outcome. This theory has proven to be effective in influencing oral hygiene in young adults. The social expectations of the group had a strong influence on their oral hygiene behavior. Applying this concept to patient education, a teenager may consistently practice oral hygiene at home, but a change in environment, such as moving to student housing at college, may change intentions and behavior. Fatigue associated with student life also might affect oral health practices.

III. The Theory of Planned Behavior

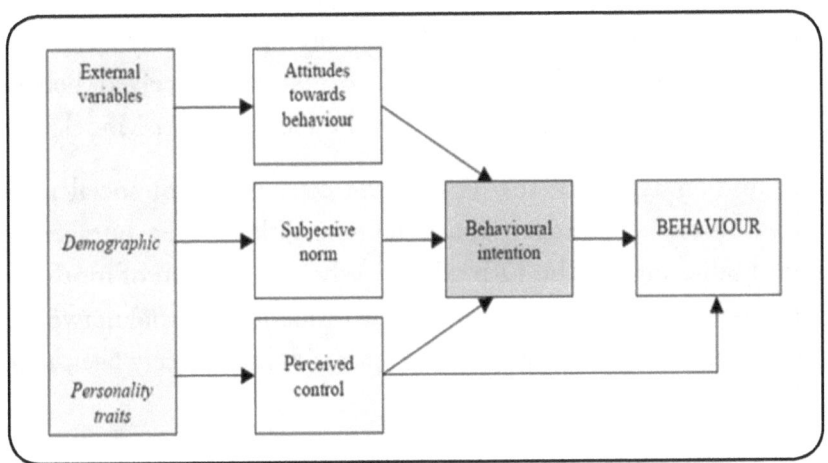

FIGURE 2

The Theory of Planned Behavior (TPB) is an extension of the earlier Theory of Reasoned Action. The theory of planned behavior center on factors which lead to a specific intention to act, or behavioral Intention in which it situates between the attitudes and behavior **(Figure 2)**. The centrality of Behavioral Intention questions the classical model of Belief, Attitude, Behavior (Conner & Sparks, 1995).[7]

In the TPB, **Behavioral Intention** is determined by:

1. **Attitudes towards behavior,** determined by the belief that a specific behavior will have a concrete consequence.

2. **Subjective norms** or **the belief** in whether other relevant persons will approve one's behavior, plus the personal motivation to fulfill with the expectations of others.

3. **Perceived behavioral control,** determined by the belief about access to the resources needed in order to act successfully, plus the perceived success of these resources (information, abilities, skills, dependence or independence from others, barriers and opportunities).

4. **Socio-demographic variables** and **personality traits** will condition attitudes, subjective norms and perceived behavioral control. These are the same as in the Health Belief Model.

An outstanding aspect of the TPB is the central role of social network support. Another key factor emphasized in the TPB is the encouragement of feelings of self-control. The TPB takes clearly into account of motivational aspects of personal disease control and the influence of social networks and peer pressure. Unfortunately, the TPB approach has scarcely been used.

Limitation

A potential overemphasis on the psychological factors, while under-valuing structural factors like limited access or availability of resources.

IV. The Health Care Utilisation Model

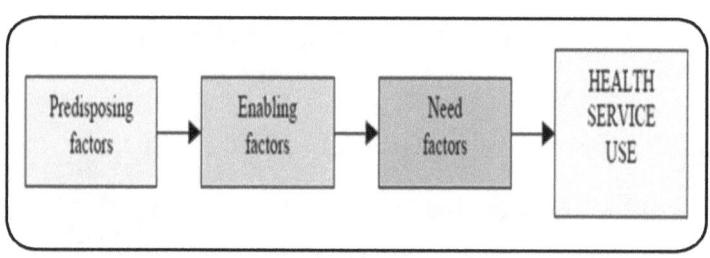

FIGURE 3

The **Socio-behavioral or Andersen model** (Andersen & Newman, 1973) groups in a logical sequence three clusters or categories of factors (predisposing, enabling and need factors) which can influence health behavior. The model was specifically developed to investigate the use of **biomedical health services.** Later versions have extended the model to include other health care sectors, i.e. traditional medicine and domestic treatments; **Figure 3** outlines the different categories. An adaptation of the model has been proposed for studying health-seeking behavior.[8]

Factors organised in the categories of the Health Care Utilisation Model **(Weller et al. 1997)**[8] are:

1. **Predisposing factors:** age, gender, religion, global health assessment, prior experiences with illness, formal education, general attitudes towards health services and knowledge about the illness.

2. **Enabling factors:** availability of services, financial resources to purchase services, health insurance and social network support.

3. **Need factors:** perception of severity, total number of sick days for a reported illness, total number of days in bed, days missed from work or school and help from outside for caring.

V. Variant of the Health Care Utilisation Model

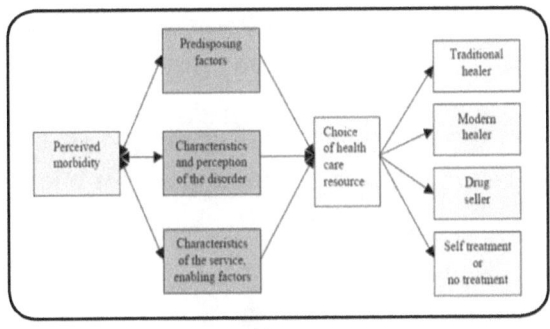

FIGURE 4

Andersen's model has been modified in the International Collaborative Study on Health Care **(Figure 4, Kroeger, 1983).** In addition to the predisposing factors and enabling factors, this version includes **Health Service System factors,** referring to the structure of the health care system and its link to a country's social and political macro-system. This is a valuable extension as it puts emphasis on the link of health-seeking behavior with structural levels within a macro-political and economic context. However, the model **omits the 'need factors'** which are central for understanding health-seeking behavior.

A further variant of Andersen's model was elaborated by **Kroeger (1983).**[9] Based on an extensive and well-elaborated literature revision, he proposed the following framework **(see figure 4):**

1. Interrelated explanatory variables, all of which are affected by **perceived morbidity.**

2. **An individual's traits or predisposing factors:** age, sex, marital status, status in the household, household size, ethnic group, degree of cultural adaptation, formal education, occupation, assets (land, livestock, cash, income) and social network interactions.

3. **Characteristics of the disorder and their perception:** chronic or acute, severe or trivial, etiological model, expected benefits or treatment (modern versus traditional) and psychosomatic versus somatic disorders.

4. **Characteristics of the service** (health service system factors and enabling factors): accessibility, appeal (opinions and attitudes towards **traditional and modern healers),** acceptability, quality, communication, costs.

5. The interaction of these factors guides the **election of health care resources** (dependent variables).

The **advantage** of socio-behavioural models is the variety of the factors which are organised in categories, making interventions on therapeutic actions (or lack of actions) feasible. They permit the establishment of correlations with good predictability, but not specification of how and why the different factors affect therapeutic selection **(Weller et al. 1997).**

VI. The "Four A's" Model

It has become popular among researchers to use different categories which group key factors for health-seeking behaviour. The best known is grouping into the "four A's" as follows:

1. **Availability:** refers to the geographic distribution of health facilities, pharmaceutical products and so on.

2. **Accessibility:** includes transport, roads and so on.

3. **Affordability:** includes treatment costs for the individual, household or family. A distinction is made between direct, indirect and opportunity costs.

4. **Acceptability:** relates to cultural and social distance. This mainly refers to the characteristics of the health providers – health workers' behaviour, gender aspects (non-acceptance of being treated by the opposite sex, in particular women who refuse to be seen by male nurses/doctors) and so on.[9]

The 'model' of the "four A's" has been widely used by medical geographers, anthropologists and epidemiologists who mainly emphasized distance (both social and geographical) and economic aspects as key factors for access to treatment.

Advantage

The easy identification of key potential 'barriers' for adequate treatment.

VII. Pathway Models

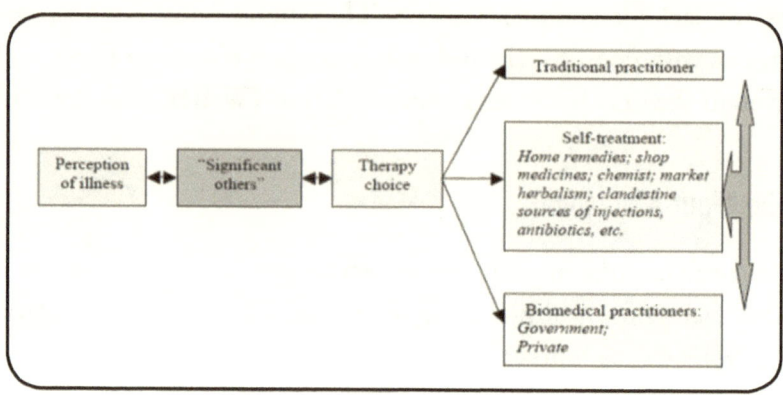

FIGURE 5

Starting with recognition of symptoms, Pathway model centres on the path that people follow until they use different health services (home treatment, traditional healer, biomedical facility). **Figure 5** shows an example of a pathway model **(Good et al 1987)**[10], which stresses the importance of 'significant others' and the decision-making process which are discussed below as follows:

'Significant others' are part of the 'therapy managing group', a concept elaborated by **Janzen (1978)** which is key for understanding decision making in therapeutic processes. This idea challenges the strong emphasis on the individual and stresses the pivotal role of extended groups of relatives and friends in illness negotiation and management. In the course of the illness episode, the involvement of support groups in illness management can successively change.

Pathway models acknowledge these **dynamics of illness and decision-making.** Most of the studies which use pathway models investigate the path until the first contact with a health facility. More recently, there has been an increasing emphasis on successive therapy choices. The **strength of pathway models** is that they depict health seeking as a dynamic process. Factors are sequentially organized, according to the different key steps (i.e. recognition of symptoms, decision making, medical encounter, evaluation of outcomes, re-interpretation of illness) which determine the course of the therapy path.

VIII. Social Cognition Models

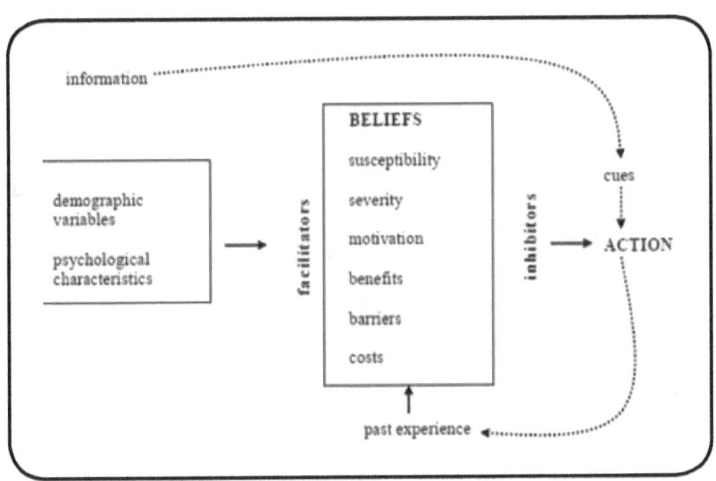

FIGURE 6

A second genre of model is linked to the general assumption that those who believe they have control over their health are more likely to engage in health promoting behaviors **(Figure 6, Normand and Bennett, 1996)**[10]. The 'health locus of control' construct is therefore utilised to assess the relationship between an individual's actions and experience from previous outcomes. The most popular of these is 'the multidimensional health locus of control measure' (Wallston, 1992). However, this approach to social cognition models has been criticized for taking too narrow an approach to health and because the amount of variance explained is low.

Other approaches, including 'protection motivation theory' and 'theory of planned behavior' have equally met with mixed reception (Boer and Seydel, 1996; Conner and Sparks, 1996). **Figure 6** represents a visual summary of the approach of social cognition models. These models, attempting to predict health behavior through a variety of means, are predicted on two assumptions central to classic health promotion: health is influenced by behavior; behavior is modifiable. The downfall of these models is that most view the individual as a rational decision maker, systematically reviewing available information and forming behavior intentions from this. They do not allow any understanding of how people make decisions, or a description of the way in which people make decisions.

Fazio (1990) proposes an alternative to this 'deliberative processing model' in the form of a 'spontaneous processing model' which takes greater account of the unpredictable nature of the actual process of decision making. However, the central problem remains that these models focus on the individual and the centrality of cognitive processes ('I know, therefore I act'). This loses the sense that we are all rooted in social contexts that affect, in a far more complex manner, the way we process and act on information.

IX. Conceptual Framework (Modified from Anderson)

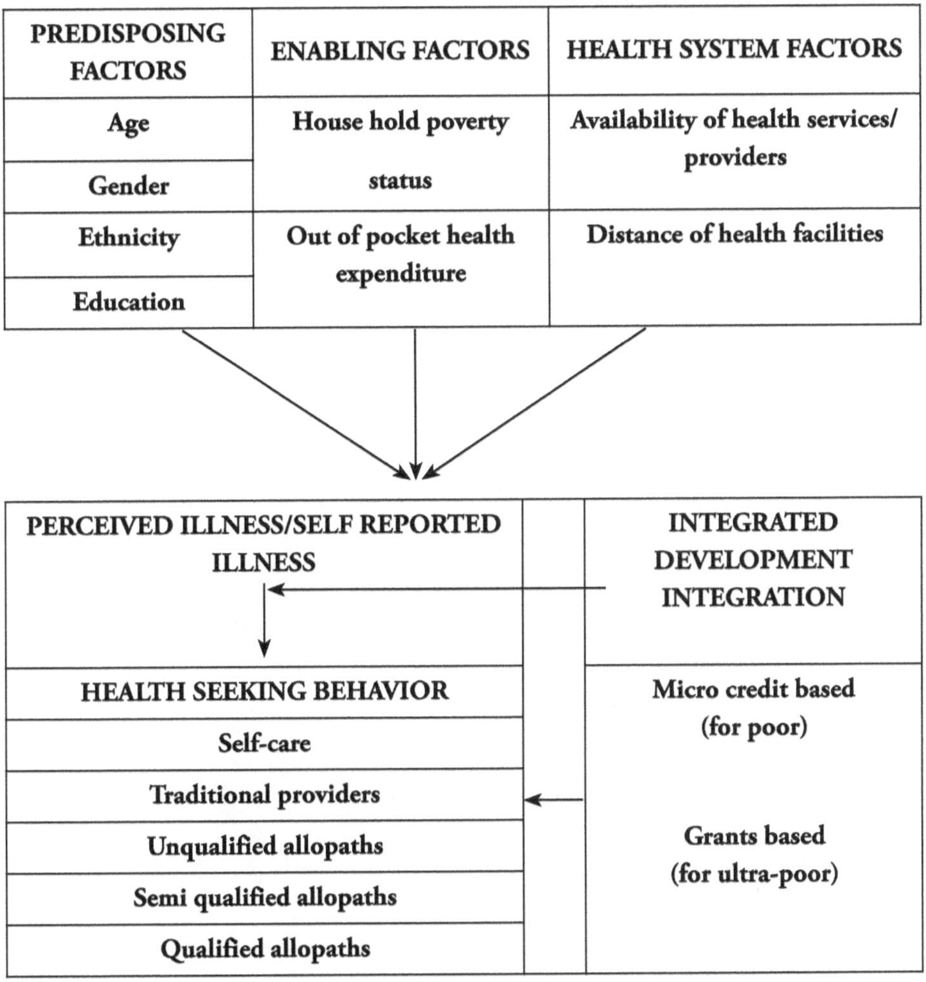

PREDISPOSING FACTORS	ENABLING FACTORS	HEALTH SYSTEM FACTORS
Age	House hold poverty status	Availability of health services/providers
Gender		
Ethnicity	Out of pocket health expenditure	Distance of health facilities
Education		

PERCEIVED ILLNESS/SELF REPORTED ILLNESS	INTEGRATED DEVELOPMENT INTEGRATION
HEALTH SEEKING BEHAVIOR	Micro credit based (for poor)
Self-care	
Traditional providers	
Unqualified allopaths	Grants based (for ultra-poor)
Semi qualified allopaths	
Qualified allopaths	

FIGURE 7

In **1973, Andersen and Newman**[8] proposed a framework for evaluating the utilization of health care. This model assumes that a person's use of health services is a function of predisposing, enabling and need factors which are described below as follows:

1. **Predisposing** characteristics include gender, marital status, educational level, occupation, length of time in the community and health beliefs. Health beliefs such as attitudes, values and knowledge of the dental care delivery system are often influenced by cultural values.

2. **Enabling resources** refer to attributes specific to the individual or the community (e.g. income, social network, access to regular source of care). Need variables reflect illness levels that require the use of services.

3. **Needs** can be perceived by the individual and are influenced by cultural beliefs and values (e.g. perceived health status, disease severity, limitation of activity).

In 1997, an expanded version of this model was developed as a conceptual framework for the WHO International Collaborative Study of Oral Health Outcomes (ICS II, **Figure 7**), which was undertaken in selected industrialized countries. This theoretical model was derived by integrating existing oral health behavior and oral health status models with the general health model of Andersen and Newman.[8]

ORAL HEALTH SEEKING BEHAVIOR MODELS

A BRIEF OVERVIEW

Behavior and perceptions are among the many factors determining oral and general health status in various populations and groups. Behavior is modifiable and provides addressable factors for health promotion efforts. Lifestyle improvement, preventive self-care behaviors and better use of formal preventive health services is among these factors. The task of analyzing the multifactorial relationships between key variables associated with oral health behaviors and perceptions is especially difficult. Models have been proposed to assist in understanding the factors associated with general and oral health seeking behavior, clinical status and satisfaction.

A variety of models are proposed to study health seeking behavior of populations. These general health seeking behavior models are being utilized in dentistry to assess the oral health related behaviors of individuals in the society. Three models which were specifically applied in various studies to understand oral health behavior which could further help in improvement of oral health status are discussed.

The three Oral health seeking behavior models are listed below:

I. Conceptual framework model by Gloria C et al, 2008.

II. Anderson's Behavioral model modified by ICS-II, USA.

III. Conceptual model for Oral and General health by Kathryn A et al, 2003.

I. Conceptual Framework Model by Gloria C Et Al, 2008

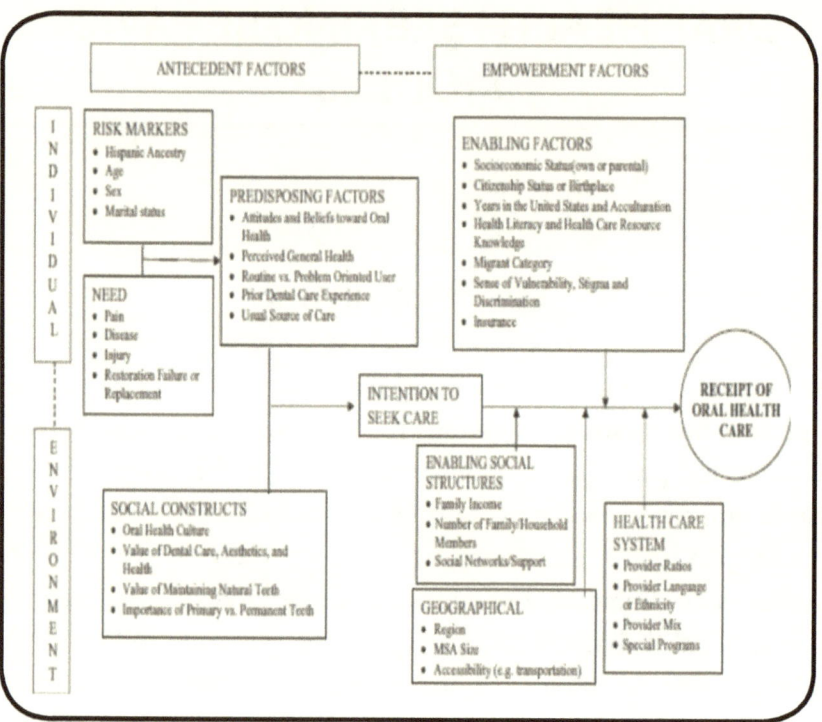

FIGURE 8

The proposed conceptual framework **(Figure 8)** considers the classic model of health service utilization by Andersen and Newman, but also takes into account the work of several other health behavior and social scientists.

Ajzen, in the "Theory of Planned Behavior," recognizes the importance of behavioral intention and introduces the concept of perceived behavioral control/empowerment. Behavioral intention is defined as the perceived likelihood of performing the behavior, and perceived behavioral control is an overall measure of the individual's perception of their ability to perform the behavior.

The Triandis model considers behavioral intention as a predictor of behavior, affected by personal and social components such as the appropriateness of performing the behavior, and adds habit and "facilitating conditions" as predictors of behavior. In the present model proposed by Gloria C et al, authors have incorporated the concept of behavioral intention through the **"intention to seek care"** domain, which is determined by individual and environmental antecedent factors. Intention then becomes a corner stone in the process of seeking and receiving care. The "Social Cognitive Theory," through its reciprocal determinism postulate, emphasizes the interactions between individuals, their behavior, and the environment. Authors argue in support of this theory on the dynamic interaction between individual and environment; however, they believe that behavior is integral and inseparable from the individual, and therefore they have not used it as a separate construct.[11]

II. Anderson's Behavioural Model Modified By ICS-II, USA

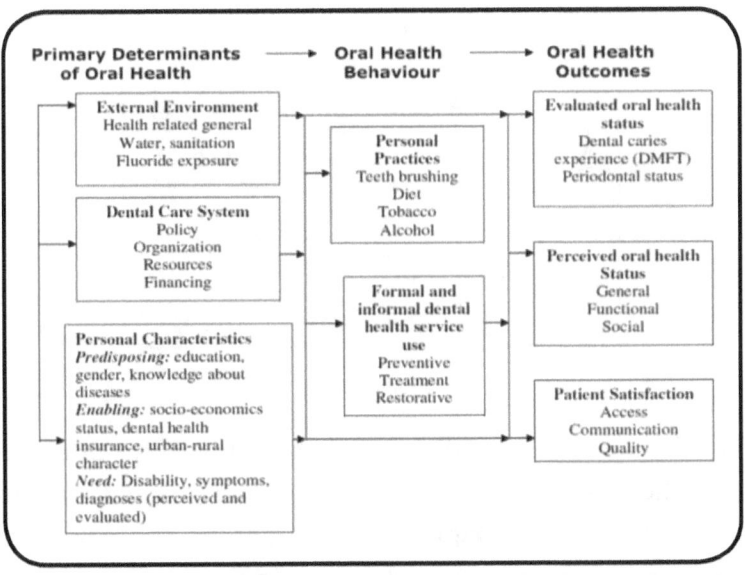

FIGURE 9

Figure 9 shows the Anderson's behavioral model of health services utilization modified by the international collaborative study for oral health outcomes[8] (ICS-II, USA).

The framework suggests that the **primary determinants of health** which are divided in characteristics of the external environment, the dental care system and the personal characteristics of the populations influence oral health behavior. At the same time, oral health behaviors are conceptualized as intermediate dependant variables that would influence the oral health outcomes (evaluated, self-perceived and patient satisfaction).

III. Conceptual Model for Oral and General Health By Kathryn a Et Al, 2003

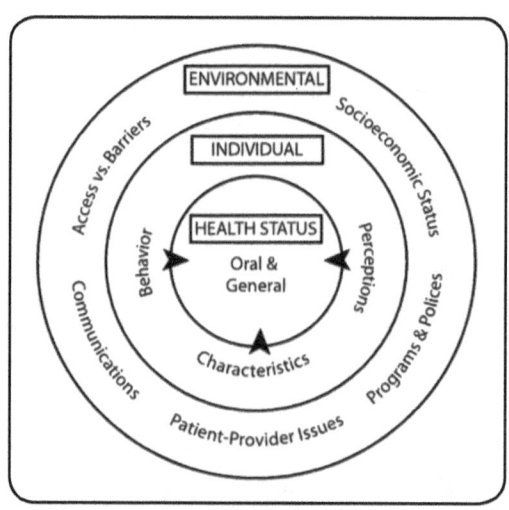

FIGURE 10

Some models focus on the individual's behavior, whereas others consider behavior in the context of community mores and program planning. The above model presented as **Figure 10** incorporates concepts from older models within conceptual framework (concentric rings surrounding health status) of dynamic interactions among the variables. **Evans and**

Stoddert proposed a model that considers individual responses to the social and physical environment, along with genetic endowment, as factors determining health and disease and, ultimately, well-being. **Andersen** presented an early model that included the individual's background and behavior as key factors in health.[12]

This Behavioral Model for Health Services Use by Katryn et al **(Figure 10)** has been updated and applied in various health settings, including oral health. In this framework, population characteristics are conceptualized as precursors to health behaviors and outcomes. **Satisfaction** is included as an outcome measure along with perceived and evaluated health status. **Demographic factors** such as age, gender, income, social structure, and beliefs are considered **"predisposing"** characteristics that interface with **"enabling"** resources in the family and community to address needs. Predictors of health behaviors, including factors related to failure to seek dental care among disadvantaged Hispanic and black adults at low cost medical and dental clinics, were analyzed by researchers at the Los Angeles Research Center for Minority Oral Health. Among other relevant findings related to personal practices and health service utilization, older age, lower education level, and less acculturation were correlated with poorer oral health status among the Hispanic participants.

Increasingly, researchers and program planners have come to recognize that understanding health behavior and community involvement are essential for program effectiveness, particularly for minority communities. The **"PRECEDE–PROCEED"** model is used for addressing the needs of targeted populations in a program planning and evaluation context. The target community is involved in needs assessment and evaluation of program goals, interventions, and progress. The health promotion framework consists of a diagnostic phase identifying predisposing, reinforcing, and enabling constructs in educational diagnosis and evaluation (acronym ¼ PRECEDE), followed by policy, regulatory, and organizational constructs in educational and environmental development (acronym ¼ PROCEED). This model was applied to an oral health promotion program in a Washington DC, inner-city Latino community. Focus groups of mothers and pregnant women were involved in the initial assessment of "predisposing" knowledge and beliefs regarding oral health and dental caries prevention. The second phase of assessment involved base-line surveys of the knowledge, opinions, and practices of preschool children and their parents. A culturally appropriate intervention program was developed based on the scientific literature, focus groups, and baseline survey results. The full-scale intervention consisted of targeted presentations and a mass-media campaign. Process evaluation throughout the program was used to refine it, whereas the overall impact and usefulness were evaluated at the end of the intervention.[12] A variety of problems, which illustrates the importance of simultaneously studying the socioeconomic and political environment, were identified, they are:-

1. Community priorities (general versus oral health, unemployment, housing, violence).

2. Competition and friction between community-based programs.

3. Funding issues and budget cuts.

CRITIQUES OF HEALTH SEEKING BEHAVIOUR MODELS

1. The studies about health-seeking behavior centre on the characteristics of the implied persons for explaining, from an applied Public Health perspective, reasons for delay in receiving adequate treatment, non-compliance with treatment, or non-utilization of preventive measures. Few models take into consideration health provider factors. Centering on the personal characteristics tends to 'blame the victim', showing the individuals themselves as responsible for inadequate health-seeking behavior. In general, they overestimate the capacity for an individual to choose and follow behavior which is considered adequately.

2. In most cases, health-seeking behavior models depart from the assumption that individuals generally aim to maximize utility and thus prefer behaviors which are associated with the highest expected benefits. This is, however, a very utilitarian vision which does not necessarily correspond to reality. Emotional aspects and non-rational behavior which influence strongly health-seeking behavior are much less considered. Decision-making issues are also manifestations of power relations which encompass interests in conflicts that go beyond the strict domain of health. Actions contain also a symbolic value, and much of behavior is determined by political and politicised discourses. Peer pressure factors and

social relations of the "Theory of Planned Behavior" to a certain extent consider these points, but they commonly understate the social forces from a more historical perspective.

3. More explicitly, the behavioral models attempt to identify key factors, and their weight in behavior. Key factors can, however, not be isolated from the context in which they occur. Sauerborn et al showed how perception of illness severity changed with seasonality, related with climatic conditions and work load.

BARRIERS AFFECTING ORAL HEALTH SEEKING BEHAVIOR

Barrier is defined as an obstacle or any condition that makes it difficult to make progress or to achieve an objective. Certain barriers to achieve good oral health still exist even after a significant progress made globally in reducing major dental diseases like caries and periodontal diseases. To provide appropriate oral health care services it is very important to first identify the barriers which are obstructing in the path of achieving a healthy life. Only after knowing about the barriers which exists in the society we could take certain actions to solve them. There are few barriers to oral health seeking behavior which are listed and enumerated below according to various authors as follows:

1. **BARRIERS TO SEEKING DENTAL SERVICES (FDI):**[13]

    a. **Individuals themselves:-**

    - Lack of perceived need.
    - Anxiety or fear.
    - Financial considerations.
    - Lack of access.

    b. **The dental profession:-**

    - Inappropriate manpower resources.
    - Uneven geographical distribution.

- Inappropriate training to changing needs and demands.
- Insufficient sensitivity to patient's attitudes and needs.

c. **Society:-**
- Insufficient public support of attitudes conducive to health.
- Inadequate oral health care facilities.
- Inadequate oral health manpower planning.
- Insufficient support for research.

2. **BARRIERS AFFECTING UTILIZATION OF DENTAL SERVICES[14]:**

   a. **The barriers under the control of the dentist are:**
   - The high cost of the treatment.
   - Inaccessibility of the service (practice).
   - The difficulty of getting an appointment when desired.
   - Restricted amount of dental services offered.
   - Dentists attitude, inexperience, way of communicating and knowledge.

   b. **Barriers related to patient characteristic are:**
   - Lack of perceived need.
   - Pain.
   - Fear.
   - Dislike.
   - Forgetfulness.

- Lack of time.
- Laziness.
- Poor expectations.
- Lack of perceived seriousness.
- Inconvenience.
- Uncooperativeness (in the case of treatment of children).

3. 'ACCESS' PROBLEMS TO DESCRIBE THE DIFFICULTIES EXPERIENCED WITH SERVICE USE[12]:

Access to health care is a complex issue, which can have two aspects.

The first aspect: Relates to factors which influence whether a person will make contact with health services. These factors have psychological and sociological explanations. Example: How culture can affect a person's response to symptoms and use of services and how people's beliefs, attitudes, exploitations and definitions of sickness can affect service use.

The second aspect: Relates to the fit between the health care service and the clients, assuming the latter have overcome cultural and psychological issues and have decided to use health care.

Various access related problems are as follows:

a. Availability of services

b. Accessibility of services

c. Affordability of services

d. Acceptability of services

e. Accommodation of services

a. **Availability of services:** This refers to how well distributed the health services are. The example includes Dentist: Population ratio in a locality. Doctors like to set up practices in middle class areas where need for such services are small. Thus there is an abundance of practices in middle class areas and a small number in more deprived areas like rural or inner city where needs are greater. In other words, health services are often located in areas where the needs are low, but in areas where the needs are greatest, few services are found. This paradox was described by Tudor–Hart as the "inverse care law'. Another consequence of the perception of the availability of services is the impact on the uptake of care. Reasons for shortage of dentists in rural areas or inner city residents include the high level of education debt by dental graduates and limited availability of loan repayment and scholarship programs. Limited scope of practice for auxiliary personnel. Changes in the dental practice acts have the potential to increase capacity and as a result, access to care. If it is perceived that services are limited then demand for care becomes suppressed.

b. **Accessibility of services:** It has two dimensions:

The first is about location:

How for you have to travel to the nearest dental practice. Example: What is the means of transport if you are not a vehicle owner?

The second aspect is a spatial dimension:

Whether a person can physically access the premises. Example: An older person with arthritis would find climbing the stairs difficult to reach a dental surgery clinic which is located in second or third floor of a building.

c. **Affordability of services:**

Payment for dental treatment can act as a barrier to people using dental services. In addition to the direct costs of dental treatment there are some indirect costs that people include in the equation about whether 'it is worth' having dental treatment.

Examples of such indirect costs are:

Having to take time off work.

Having to pay travel costs.

Some groups will suffer greater disadvantage depending on how they are paid. Low income workers are usually paid by hour, and the cost to them of taking time off work is greater than to someone on a salary.

d. **Acceptability of services:**

Users and providers of health services have expectations about how services should look and be. These expectations are not always shared.

Providers want to attract to their practice, wants patients to speak the language doctors know, patients pay on time after receiving treatment, patients behave well in the waiting room which would enhance the image of the practice.

Users would like to be made to feel welcome in the practice, feel information was easy to find, would like to be dealt with professionally but treated as an individual.

The acceptability of patients to a practice is an important issue: a dental study of homeless people in London found that they would rather use an older, shabbier dental hospital than the newly built more local dental hospital, because they perceived that older hospital was more accepting of their appearance and circumstances.

e. **Accommodation:**

This refers to the ways in which care is provided in terms of opening hours, emergency visits, late night clinics, waiting times and case of getting an appointment.

The Penchansky and Thomas framework is very useful for identifying the structural problems in the organization of health care, but it ignores the behavioural science explanation of access.

4. BARRIERS TO THE RECEIPT OF DENTAL CARE (FINCH ET AL, 1988)[15]

The terms 'access to care' and 'barriers to care' are both used in the literature, but essentially mean the same thing. In 1985 Finch examined the reasons why people did not use dental services regularly, and he used the term 'barriers to the receipt of dental care'.

a. **Main barriers:**

- Fear of dental treatment.
- Cost of dental treatment.

b. **Other barriers:**

- Reception and waiting room procedures.
- Personality of the dentist.
- Small clinic with lack of adequate space.
- Hearing the sounds of dental treatment.
- White coats and bright lights.
- Feeling vulnerable in dental chair.
- Travel time.
- Time off work.

5. BARRIERS TO DENTAL CARE (LENNON ET AL, 1988):

Access to dental services can be restricted due to financial, political and emotional barriers or a combination of any two of these.

a. **Financial barriers:**

   Low income can result in several disadvantages.

   Family which is struggling financially has difficulty in paying fees, and also finding the money for bus fares.

   Self employed people might have to forego earnings to visit a dentist.

b. **Physical barriers:**

   Dentists can establish their practices wherever they like and this has led to an uneven distribution of services. Majority of practices are clustered in the more affluent areas, thus making a dental visit more difficult for those patients relying on public transport.

   Leichter (1980) identified three major problems in service provision:

   i. There is an uneven geographical distribution of resources.

   ii. There are fewer health care resources in poor areas than affluent ones.

   iii. Many priorities are determined on political and professional grounds and are derived from the way that health care is socially organized.

   Example: There is more money available for acute specialties than for patients with chronic problems which require long term care.

c. **Emotional barriers:**

   Dentistry has the reputation of being painful and it seems that some people are reluctant to visit a dentist because they expect to experience pain.

Smith and Sheiham's (1980) study of elderly people showed that people who would have liked to receive treatment had not tried to obtain it because they felt they were 'too old', while many who were in pain who did not want to 'waste the dentist's time'. These feelings of low personal worth and that dental care is not 'worth it' may be important barriers for many elderly people.

6. BARRIERS TO HEALTH SEEKING BEHAVIOR AMONG WOMEN (NASH OJANUGA AND GILBERT, 1992)[16]:

a. **Institutional barriers:** Unequal treatment by health providers.

b. **Economic barriers:** Different access to resources.

c. **Cultural barriers:** Social status of women which situates them in socially inferior positions, male doctors attend women with sensitive health problems.

d. **Education barriers:** Women having less access to education.

According to center for dental service studies, 1998 lack of information and openness continued to be a common complaint about dental care in the UK, and there appeared lack of trust between dentists and patients. The reasons are given for appropriate use of services as follows:

The appropriate use of health services is a complex issue. People may have very valid reasons for using services in a way that health professionals may not advise. This may arise due to lay and health professional communication problems.

Lay people have different expectations and different concepts of health, their use of health services will reflect these differences.

Example: Consider the issue of regular attendance at the dentist. Advice over the years has been regular attendance every 6 months.

But given the decline in decay rates amongst young people, this is no longer an appropriate recommendation. As people become more aware of oral health issues many are choosing not to attend regularly, because they know from past experience they need very little oral health care. Guidance on what is regular attendance must depend on the individual, their oral health problems, and their life circumstances.

Many different groups in societies have difficulties in accessing dental services. Most of these groups have diverse problems which bring about disadvantage, but what they do share is a common experience of access problems.

A DIAGRAMATIC REPRESENTATION OF BARRIERS TO HEALTH SEEKING BEHAVIOR

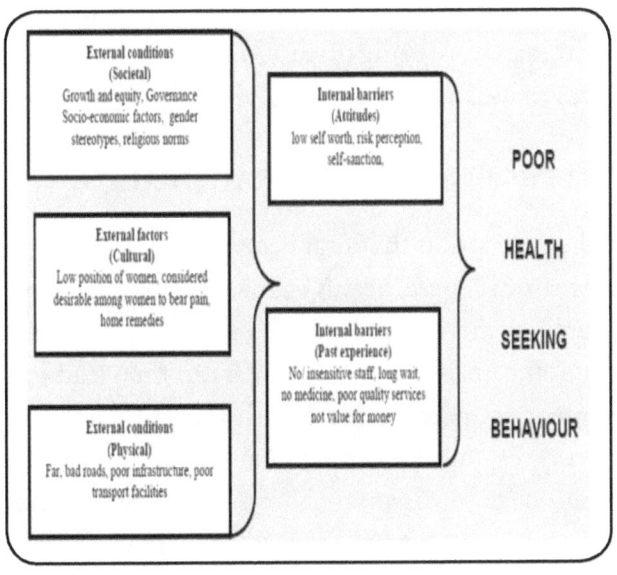

OVERCOMING BARRIERS TO ORAL HEALTH SEEKING BEHAVIOR

Despite considerable progress in oral health care achieved in recent years, dental caries as well as periodontal diseases remain the most common chronic diseases. With a rapid universal increase in the growth of the population there is an increased oral health care needs of the population. A very challenging task is to maintain utmost health of individuals and populations. The recognition that oral health is a critical component of holistic health appears rather more challenging than maintaining general health. Several strategies are being discussed below to improve the utilization of dental services as well as to improve oral health seeking behavior:-

1. CHANGE PERCEPTIONS OF ORAL HEALTH

For too long, the perception that oral health is in some way less important than and separate from general health has been deep-rooted in consciousness of people throughout the world. Activities to overcome these attitudes and beliefs can start at the grassroots level, which can then lead to a coordinated national movement to increase oral health literacy. Oral health literacy is defined as the degree to which individuals have the capacity to obtain, process, and understand basic oral and craniofacial information and services needed to make appropriate health decisions.

By raising level of awareness and understanding of oral health, people can make informed decisions and articulate their expectations of what they, their communities and oral health professionals can contribute to improving health. Health professionals and researchers can benefit from work with oral health partners; and policymakers can commit to including oral health in health policies. In this way, the prevention, early detection, and management of diseases of the dental, oral, and craniofacial tissues can become integrated in health care, community-based programs, and social services, and promote overall health and well-being.[17]

Implementation strategies to change perceptions are needed at local, state, regional, and national levels and for all population groups. All stakeholders should work together and use data in order to:

Change public perceptions

    a. Enhance oral health literacy.

    b. Develop messages that are culturally sensitive and linguistically competent.

    c. Enhance knowledge of the value of regular, professional oral health care.

    d. Increase the understanding of how the signs and symptoms of oral infections can indicate general health status and act as a marker for other diseases.

Change policymakers' perceptions

    a. Inform policymakers and administrators at local, state, and federal levels of the results of oral health research and programs and of the oral health status of their constituencies.

    b. Develop concise and relevant messages for policymakers.

    c. Document the health and quality-of-life outcomes that result from the inclusion (or exclusion) of oral health services in programs and reimbursement schedules.

Change health providers' perceptions

a. Review and update health professional educational curricula and continuing education courses to include content on oral health and the association between oral health and general health.

b. Train health care providers to conduct oral screenings as part of routine physical exams and make appropriate referrals.

c. Promote interdisciplinary training of medical, oral health, and allied health professional personnel in counseling patients about how to reduce risk factors common to oral and general health.

d. Encourage oral health providers to refer patients to other health specialists as warranted by examinations and history. Similarly, encourage medical and surgical providers to refer patients for oral health care when medical or surgical treatments that may impact oral health are planned.[18]

2. OVERCOME BARRIERS BY REPLICATING EFFECTIVE PROGRAMS AND ESTABLISHED/PROVEN EFFORTS

Reduce disease and disability

The effectiveness of preventive interventions such as community water fluoridation and school-based dental sealants applied to children at risk have been convincingly demonstrated. Several projects and demonstration programs are conducted by research workers to inform the public and health professionals on ways to reduce the burden of oral disease through education, behavior change, risk reduction, early diagnosis, and disease prevention management. Local efforts to engage and educate community leaders in activities to improve oral health have been developed. The designs and outcomes of those programs should be well documented, evaluated, and made available to others. *The Guides to Community Preventive Service and The Guides to Clinical Preventive Services* provide criteria and strong foundations for evaluating the scientific evidence and promoting effective interventions.

Having accurate data on disease and disabilities for a given population is critical. Program success depends on how well the program is designed and implemented to address the defined problems. While available data reveal variations within and among states and population groups in patterns of health and disease, there are many subpopulations for which data are limited or nonexistent.

Improve oral health care access

Health disparities are commonly associated with populations whose access to health care services is compromised by poverty, limited education or language skills, geographic isolation, age, gender, disability, or an existing medical condition. Public dental insurance plans have not completely closed the gap in access problems. Adults lacking language skills or reading competence may not know that they or their children are eligible for dental (or medical) services.

Those who seek care may be faced with health practitioners who lack the training and cultural competence to communicate effectively in order to provide needed services. Programs that have overcome these barriers, including outreach efforts and community service activities conducted through dental schools and other health professional schools and residency programs, should be highlighted and replicated.

Compounding health disparity problems is the lack of adequate reimbursement for oral care services in both public and private programs. Private insurance coverage for dental care is in its preliminary stage and still lags behind medical insurance. Inadequate reimbursement has been reported for many Medicaid and SCHIP programs in western countries. Outreach programs could be conducted in communities and provider participation could be improved through operational changes. These improvements include increasing dental reimbursement to competitive levels, eliminating technical administrative barriers and modeling commercial insurance programs. The federal effort to address gaps in care through new funding for oral health services at Community Health Centers and primary Health Centers is also a positive step.[19]

Enhance health promotion and health literacy

Public policies and community interventions to make health care and information more accessible have been effective. Efforts should be made to encourage healthier lifestyles and increase interventions for prevention or early detection of disease by changing the environment (the places where people work, play, learn, or live). Expansion of community-based health promotion and disease prevention programs, including increasing understanding of what individuals can do to enhance oral health, is essential if the needs of the public are to be met. Policies and programs concerning tobacco cessation, dietary choices, wearing protective gear for sports, and other lifestyle-related efforts not only will benefit oral health, but are natural ways to integrate oral health promotion with promotion of general health and well-being.

Several oral health campaigns should be organized for raising awareness of why oral health is important and how to access care, such as nationwide campaigns. It is encouraging that messages like these are being communicated—through public service announcements and campaigns. Mass media, electronic media, bill boards, web services and television could be utilized as best resources to spread the message about importance of oral health. More needs to be done in this direction to increase the health literacy of the public.

3. BUILD THE SCIENCE BASE AND ACCELERATE SCIENCE TRANSFER

Advances in health depend on biomedical and behavioral research aimed at understanding the causes and pathological processes of diseases. Not much emphasis is laid on health services research which is as important as other two researches namely biomedical and behavioral research. This can lead to interventions that will improve prevention, diagnosis, and treatment. Too many people outside the oral health community are uninformed about, misinformed about, or simply not interested in oral health. Such lack of understanding and indifference may explain why community water fluoridation and school-based dental sealant programs fall short of full implementation, even though the scientific evidence for their effectiveness has been known since some time. These and other effective preventive and early detection programs should be expanded—especially to populations at risk.

Biomedical and behavioral research in the 21st century will provide the knowledge base for health care practice. This scientific foundation requires the support of the full range of research from basic studies to large-scale clinical trials. To achieve a balanced science collection, it is essential to expand clinical studies, especially the study of complex oral diseases that involve the interactions of genetic, behavioral, and environmental factors. Clinical trials are needed to test interventions to diagnose and manage oral infections, complications from systemic diseases and their treatment, congenital and acquired defects, and other conditions. Oral health research must also pursue research on chronic oral infections associated with heart and lung disease, diabetes, and premature low-birth-weight babies. Such research must be complemented by prevention and behavioral science research (including community-based approaches and ways to change risk behavior), health services research to explore how the structure and function of health care services affect health outcomes, and by population health and epidemiology research to understand potential associations among diseases and possible risk factors. Surveys are needed to establish baseline health data as well as to monitor changing patterns of disease.

No one can predict the findings from genetic studies in the years ahead, but without question these advances will profoundly affect health, even indicating an individual's susceptibility to major diseases and disorders. Hybrid sciences of importance to oral health are also on the rise. For example, bioengineering studies are establishing the basis for repair and regeneration of the body's tissues and organs—including teeth, bones, and joints—and ultimately full restoration of function. Oral diagnostics, using saliva or oral tissue samples, will contribute to overall health surveillance and monitoring.

If the public and their care providers are to benefit from research, efforts are needed to transfer new oral knowledge into improved means of diagnosis, treatment, and prevention. The public need clear descriptions of the results from research and demonstration projects concerning lifestyle behaviors and disease prevention practices. At the same time, research is needed to determine the effect of oral health literacy on oral health. Communities and organizations must also be able to gather the benefits of scientific advances, which may contribute to changes in the reimbursement and delivery of services, as well as enhance knowledge of risk factors. Advances in science and technology also mean that life-long learning for practitioners is essential, as is open lines of communication among laboratory scientists, clinicians, and the academic faculties that design the curricula, write the textbooks, and teach the classes that prepare the next generation of health care providers.[20]

Implementation strategies to build a balanced science base and accelerate science transfer should benefit all consumers, especially those in poorest oral health or at greatest risk. Specifically, there is a need to:

Enhance **applied research** (clinical and population-based studies, demonstration projects, health services research) to improve oral health and prevent disease.

   a. Expand intervention studies aimed at preventing and managing oral infections and complex diseases, including new approaches to prevent dental caries and periodontal diseases.

   b. Intensify population-based studies aimed at the prevention of oral cancer and oral-facial trauma.

   c. Conduct studies to elucidate potential underlying mechanisms and determine any causal associations between oral infections and systemic conditions. If associations are demonstrated, test interventions to prevent or lower risk of complications.

   d. Develop diagnostic markers for disease susceptibility and progression of oral diseases.

   e. Develop and test diagnostic tools for oral diseases that can be used in research and in practice.

   f. Investigate risk assessment approaches for individuals and communities, and translate them into optimal prevention, diagnosis, and treatment measures.

   g. Develop biologic measures of disease and health that can be used as outcome variables and applied in epidemiologic studies and clinical trials.

   h. Develop reliable and valid measures of patients' oral health outcomes for use in programs and in practice.

   i. Support research on the effectiveness of community-based and clinical interventions.

j. Facilitate collaborations among health professional schools, state health programs, patient groups, professional associations, private practitioners, industries, and communities to support the conduct of clinical and community-based research as well as accelerate science transfer.

Accelerate the effective transfer of science into public health and private practice

   a. Promote effective disease prevention measures that are underutilized.

   b. Routinely transfer oral health research findings to health professional school curricula and continuing education programs and incorporate appropriate curricula from other health professions-medical, nursing, pharmacy, and social work in to dental education.

   c. Communicate research findings to the public, clearly describing behaviors and actions that promote health and well-being.

   d. Explore ways to accelerate the transfer of research findings into delivery systems, including appropriate changes in reimbursement for care.

   e. Routinely evaluate the scientific evidence and update care recommendations.

4. INCREASE ORAL HEALTH WORKFORCE DIVERSITY, CAPACITY AND FLEXIBILITY:

Meet patient needs:

Patients usually accept a dental practitioner who belongs to the same community or of a culture similar to that of patients. As such, the provider can play a catalytic role as a community spokesperson, addressing key health problems and service needs. While the number of women engaged in the health professions is increasing, the number of underrepresented racial and ethnic minorities is decreasing and remains limited. Specific racial and ethnic groups are underrepresented in the active dental profession compared to their representation in the general population. The reasons for under representation of such groups are complex but certainly include the high cost of dental school education. Efforts to address these problems at all levels—from improving Kindergarten to twelve education in science to providing scholarships and loan forgiveness programs for college and pre-doctoral programs—are essential if a truly representative health workforce is to be achieved. Efforts require full community participation, mentorship, and creative outreach as well as building upon federal or state legislation and programs.

Enhance oral health workforce capacity:

Dentists are significantly under represented within rural areas, especially in smaller and more isolated locations. Dental school recruitment programs that offer incentives to students who may want to return to practice in rural areas and inner cities are in a prime position to act. Through these programs schools increase the diversity of the oral health workforce. To effect change in oral health workforce capacity, more training and recruitment efforts are needed. The lack of personnel with oral health expertise at all levels in public health programs remains a serious problem, as does the projected unmet oral health faculty and researcher needs. In public health programs, oral health professionals are needed to implement surveillance, assess needs, and target population-based preventive programs. Oral health professionals in state health agencies frequently promote integration of federal, state, and local strategies and serve as the linking agent for public-private collaborations. Currently, there is an acknowledged crisis in the ability to recruit faculty to dental schools and to attract clinicians into research careers. Dental school faculty and oral health researchers are needed to address the various scientific challenges and opportunities oral health presents, and to help transfer emerging knowledge to the next generation of health care providers. The lack of trained professionals ultimately results in a loss in the public's health. Scholarships and loan forgiveness program could make a difference, but more public investment in developing health workforce personnel is needed.

Enhance flexibility and develop local solutions:

The movement of some states towards more flexible laws, including licensing experienced dentists by qualifications is a positive one. State practice act changes that would permit, for example, alternative models of delivery of needed care for underserved populations, such as low-income children or institutionalized persons, would allow a more flexible and efficient workforce. Further, all health care professionals, whether trained at privately or publicly supported medical, dental, or allied health professional schools, need to be enlisted in local efforts to eliminate health disparities. These activities could include participating in state-funded programs for reducing disparities, part-time service in community clinics or in health care shortage areas, assisting in community-based surveillance and health assessment activities, participating in school-based disease prevention efforts, and volunteering in health-promotion and disease-prevention efforts such as tobacco cessation programs. There is a limited scope of practice for dental auxiliaries, hence changes in the dental practice acts have the potential to increase capacity and as a result, access to care.[21]

Implementation strategies to increase diversity, capacity, and flexibility must be applied to all components of the workforce: research, education, and both private and public health administration and practice. Efforts are needed to:

Change the racial and ethnic composition of the workforce to meet patient and community needs

a. Document the outcomes of existing efforts to diversify the workforce in practice, education, and research.

b. Develop ways to expand and build upon successful recruitment and retention programs, and develop and test new programs that focus on individuals from underrepresented groups.

c. Document the outcomes of existing efforts to recruit individuals into careers in oral health education, research, and public and private health practice.

d. Create and support programs that inform and encourage individuals to pursue health and science career options in high school and during graduate years.

Ensure a sufficient workforce pool to meet health care needs

a. Expand scholarships and loan repayment efforts at all levels.

b. Specify and identify resources for conducting outreach and recruitment.

c. Develop mentoring programs to ensure retention of individuals who have been successfully recruited into oral health careers.

d. Facilitate collaborations among professional, government, academic, industry, community organizations, and other institutions that are addressing the needs of the oral health workforce.

e. Provide training in communication skills and cultural competence to health care providers and students.

Secure an adequate and flexible workforce

a. Assess the existing capacity and distribution of the oral health workforce.

b. Study how to extend or expand workforce capacity and productivity to address oral health in health care shortage areas.

c. Work to ensure oral health expertise is available to health departments and to federal, state, and local government programs.

d. Determine the effects of flexible licensure policies and state practice acts on health care access and oral health outcomes.

5. INCREASE COLLABORATIONS:

The private sector and public sector each has unique characteristics and strengths. Linking the two can result in a creative synergy for growth and development of health sector. In addition, efforts are needed within each sector to increase the capacity for program development, for building partnerships for health programs. A sustained effort is needed to build the nation's oral health infrastructure to ensure that all sectors of society—the public, private practitioners, and federal and state government personnel—have sufficient knowledge, expertise, and resources to design, implement, and monitor oral health programs. Leadership for successfully directing and guiding public agency oral health units is essential. Further, incentives must be in place for partnerships to form and flourish.

Disease prevention and health promotion campaigns and programs that affect oral and general health—such as tobacco control, diet counseling, health education aimed at pregnant women and new mothers, and support for use of oral facial protection for sports—can benefit from collaborations among public health and health care practicing communities. Interdisciplinary care is needed to manage the general health-oral health interface. Achieving and maintaining oral health requires individual action, complemented by professional care and community-based activities. Many programs require the combined efforts of social service, education, and health care services at state and local levels. Most importantly, the public in the form of voluntary organizations, community groups, or as individuals, must be included in any partnership that addresses oral and general health.

Implementation strategies to enhance partnering are key to all strategies in the Call to Action. Successful partnering at all levels of society will require efforts to:

a. Invite patient advocacy groups to lead efforts in partnering for programs directed towards their constituencies.

b. Strengthen the networking capacity of individuals and communities to address their oral health needs.

c. Incorporate views and expertise of all stakeholders and that are tailored to specific populations, conditions, or programs.

d. Strengthen collaborations among dental, medical, and public health communities for research, education, care delivery, and policy development.

e. Develop partnerships that are community-based, cross-disciplinary, and culturally sensitive.

f. Work with the Partnership Network to address the four actions previously described: change perceptions, overcome barriers, build a balanced science base, and increase oral health workforce diversity, capacity, and flexibility.

g. Evaluate and report on the progress and outcomes of partnership efforts.[21]

The Need for Action Plans with Monitoring and Evaluation Components

Activities proposed to advance any or all of the actions described above must incorporate schemes for planning and evaluation, coordination, and accountability. Because planning and evaluation are key elements in the design and implementation of any program, the need to create oral health action plans is emphasized.

Whether individuals are moved to act as volunteers in a community program, as members of a health voluntary or patient advocacy organization, employees in a private or public health agency, or health professionals at any level of research, education, or practice, the essential first step is to conduct a needs assessment and develop an oral health plan. A detailed plan is necessary to guide collaboration on the many specific actions necessary for enhancing oral health, integration of key components into the state's general health plan will assure that oral health is included where appropriate in other state health initiatives.

At any level, formal plans with goals, implementation steps, strong evaluation components, and monitoring plans will facilitate setting realistic timelines, guidelines, and budgets. The oral health plan will serve as a blueprint, one that can be a tool for enlisting collaborators and partners and attracting funding sources to ensure sustainability. Building this plan into existing health programs will maximize the integration of oral health into general health programs—not only by incorporating the expertise of multidisciplinary professional teams, but also allowing the plan to benefit from economies of scale by adding on to existing facilities, utilizing existing data and management systems, and serving the public at locations already known to patients.

To Facilitate Establishing, Monitoring and Revising Written Plans and Ensure Their Progress:

a. Align plan priorities with the views and expertise of primary stakeholders.

b. Build upon existing plans within your organization, state, or local community or apply aspects of plans established at other locations to suit program needs.

c. Ensure that cultural sensitivity is utilized in the design, development, implementation, and evaluation of plans.

d. Emphasize the value of incorporating oral health into general health plans by educating the public, health professionals, and policymakers about oral health and its relation to general health and well-being.

e. Integrate existing oral health plans into general health plans.

f. Establish and maintain a strong surveillance and evaluation effort.

g. Regularly report on progress to all stakeholders and policymakers.

h. Commit resources to ensure that oral health programs and systems include staff with sufficient time, expertise, and information systems, and address oral health needs.

FACTORS AFFECTING HEALTH SEEKING BEHAVIOR

Oral Health seeking behavior and the use of dental services is not spread evenly over the population. The variations in dental service utilization by demographic and other variables provide some basis for predicting how dental services may be used in the future. Various factors affecting health seeking behavior and utilization of dental services are listed as follows:

1. Age
2. Gender
3. Place of residence and geographic location
4. Education
5. Income
6. Occupation
7. Dental Insurance
8. Social class or Socioeconomic status
9. Environmental factors
10. Social-Psychological factors
11. Race and ethnicity
12. Socio-Cultural factors

13. Acculturation

14. Traditional healers

15. General health

16. Public private partnership

17. Organizational factors

18. Other factors

1. AGE:

Dental utilization rates are lowest for children under 5 years of age and persons over 65 years of age. The peak ages for dental visits have traditionally been the late teenage years and early adulthood, with a gradual tailing-off with increasing age. The distribution of dental service use is also the converse of how physician service are used, for use of physician services is highest among the youngest and the oldest, giving rise to the U-shaped utilization curve. The utilization patterns of dental services follow an **"inverse U-shape"** curve – low utilization rates for children under 5 years of age, a sharp, increase to the peak rates for young people between the ages of 6–24; a gradual decline in rates to the age of 65; and a sharp drop to low rates for persons aged 65 and older according to Newman and Anderson et al, 1972. The patterns of dental service utilization are a reflection of the natural history of dental disease. In part, these lower utilization rates can be explained by the number of teeth at risk to dental diseases. Young children have 20 deciduous teeth, and from 6 to 12 years of age experience a gradual transition from zero to 28 permanent teeth.

The natural history of dental disease can also help to explain the utilization rates for the population aged 5–64 years. The occurrence of dental caries becomes a reality almost as soon as teeth are present in the mouth. The need for treatment of permanent teeth is reflected in the age group 5–14 by a sharp rise in percent of population with dental visits per person/years as compared to the under 5 age group. The continued incidence of caries covers this higher rate of utilization until around the age of 35 years when most tooth surfaces have been filled or teeth have been extracted. The utilization rate does not decrease substantially at this time, however because the effects of untreated periodontal disease begin to determine need for treatment. The gradual decline in utilization rates to age 65 are most likely attributed to the growing number of missing teeth per person. The peak utilization rates occur for persons in the 5–24 years age group who experience a high incidence of caries and the beginning stages of periodontal disease. This pattern of utilization by age is consistent, even though minor variations do occur, when controlling for sex, income, race, education, place of residence and geographic region. Therefore, it is possible to say that age is an independent factor in determining utilization of dental services.[22]

The prevalence of children's utilisation of dental services varied between 60% and 34% in 1984, and between 42% and 30% in 1996 in Nordic countries. Children's use of dental services decreased significantly in four of the five Nordic countries between the mid-1980s and the mid-1990s. The main finding of the study was a marked decrease in the use of dental services by children between 1984 and 1996 in all Nordic countries except Finland.[23] This finding was in contrast to a report of increased use of general practitioner services in the Nordic countries during the same time period.[24]

The expectation of continuing global population ageing, increasing oral and dental health needs of older people, the challenge of 'maintaining maximum individual and population health', and the recognition that 'oral health is a critical component of holistic health', the provision of dental care for older people is vitally important. The population of older people is increasing both in absolute numbers and relative to the rest of the population. It is recognised that 'demographic, social, economic and political factors' influence the demand for, and supply of, care services. Older age group may be considered in three age-bands, young old (65–74), older old (75–84), and oldest (85 years and over), although that their physical and chronological age may not be the same. The majority of older people (95%) live in the community with only about 5% living in care homes. Uptake of dental care amongst older people is poor, both locally and nationally. National Health Service [NHS] data from March 2006 show that the uptake of NHS dental care is highest amongst middle-aged adults and declines with increasing age, with estimated registration rates falling from 56% in the 45–54 year age-band down to 29% amongst adults 75 years and over, in Lambeth. Similar figures are reported for Southwark (54% down to 30%) and Lewisham (58% down to 35%). Barriers to dental care amongst adults in general have been well recognized as a result of the work of Finch et al, during the 1980's and subsequent national surveys.[25]

Dental attendance amongst older people is strongly associated with having some natural teeth, higher social class, and inversely associated with fear. There has been some research into the factors which impact on uptake of dental care amongst older people in the USA and within Europe. Thirty-nine older people and/or their carers participated in focus groups. **Active barriers** to dental care in older people fell into five main categories: cost, fear, availability, accessibility and characteristics of the dentist. Lack of perception of a need for dental care was a common **'passive barrier'** amongst denture wearers in particular. The cost of dental treatment, fear of care and perceived availability of dental services emerged to influence significantly dental attendance. Older people appeared to place greater significance on system and societal change than personal action. Appropriate management of older people should be done by clinicians, policy change to address charges; consideration of when, where and how dental care is provided; and clear information for older people and their careers on available local dental services, dental charges and care pathways.[26]

2. GENDER:

The effects of gender inequalities can be clearly seen when access of women to both preventive and therapeutic measures is significantly lower compared to men for general health related diseases. For example, different studies show an increased number of male patients who attend medical services in areas where disease rates are practically the same for both sexes.[14] In general inequality in access is associated with the finding that women have to overcome more obstacles to reach treatment. In some cases, the health providers attend to men and boys better than women and girls. This behaviour is the extreme consequence of sexism among many physicians who tend to treat women's problems as less important – with the exception of reproductive health, an area which is increasingly medicalised.[14] The often disrespectful treatment and the poor quality of information which women receive lead both to poor comprehension of actions to take and to unsatisfied women who increasingly abstain from health services.

Decisions which economically affect the household lie with the breadwinner who is mostly male, making women dependent on men for accessing health services for themselves and their children. Several studies pointed to the paradox that while women as the main caretakers are the first in perceiving illness in their children, they often lack the means to adequately act because they depend on the men who control funds. While nearly all studies focus on how gender inequalities negatively affect women's health, some investigate also the situation of men. It has been pointed out that men not only have often higher labour risks than women, but also those certain other risk behaviours. Contrary to general health, utilization of dental services are more among Women as compared to Males.[14]

Women report using dental services more than men do in studies conducted among various countries. This finding is so consistent over time and so constant in all countries that have studied the issue, that it seems virtually universal – one of the few issues of which we can say it 'always' happens. It is not easy to say why women use dental services more; numerous attempts to explore the issue have not come up with convincing explanations. Self-importance has been suggested as a reason. But the trend is seen across a wide variety of cultures. However when controlled for other factors variation from the basic pattern occurs. Males and females aged 14–24 years old and those belonging to families where the head of the household had gone to college, had the same utilization rates according to Newman and Anderson, 1972, as did persons over the age of 65 years.

According to **Newman and Gift**, individuals with resources in the form of finances and education, and a positive attitude toward oral health, had the greatest probability of having a regular pattern of preventive care. The finding that self-care (e.g. brushing and flossing with recommended frequencies and using a mouthrinse) was also significantly associated with seeking preventive visits suggests that those who were more aware of the importance of prevention were also more willing to seek professional preventive appointments to increase/strengthen the effects of their self-care.[27] This may reflect the importance of dental and oral hygiene education given during dental visits. The self-care was found to be practiced more frequently among females than males is a universal phenomenon. On the other hand, the finding that females were less likely to visit a dentist for preventive reasons than males might seem surprising at first, especially as in the other studies, females visited the dentist more regularly than males. This finding may be related to the higher prevalence of dental fear reported by females in the study.[28, 29–31]

Each individuals have their own barriers to seeking preventive care. **Lack of time** is considered the most common barrier. **Fear** is considered as the other most common barrier, followed by the assumption that dental care is necessary only if pain occurs. Females reported fear more often as a barrier than males in a study.[32]

3. PLACE OF RESIDENCE AND GEOGRAPHIC LOCATION:

Proportionately more persons in urban than in rural areas visit the dentist, and the urbanites visit more regularly (NHS data and Anderson and Newman 1972). Residents in the northeast US have the highest utilization rates and residents in the south have the lowest rates perhaps due to unfavorable dentist: population ratio.

Utilization of services also varies with the size of the community; the larger the community the greater the utilization rate and smaller the community the less likely the treatment would be (McFarlane, 1965). The differences in utilization may be due to the difficulty of getting to the services and introduces barriers related to transportation. In Uganda, the number of visits to a hospital varied according to the distance of the patient's home from the hospital. Persons living within 2 miles made five visits (Jolly and King, 1970) 4 miles made 1.3 visits, 12 miles made 0.1 visits annually. These differences in utilization can also be related to SES, dental insurance, race/ethnicity and perhaps also to age and dentate status.[33]

4. EDUCATION:

The utilization rate increases with increase in the level of education and education level of the head of the household is an important predictor of how frequently the family members will utilize dental services according to Anderson and Newman, 1972 and Salber EJ et al, 1976. Young and Striffler in their evaluation of NHS data found that education and income were related independently to the frequency of dental care habits. Even when income was held constant, utilization varied proportionally to the amount of education attained by the family head. The close association between use of dental services and educational level is obvious (in the US, 1989). The majority of edentulous people, and those without dental insurance, are in the lower educational attainment groups. These factors could be influencing the use of dental services. More education and income may lead people to demand a higher standard of oral health and enable them to obtain it according to Davier AR et al, 1985.

5. INCOME:

Income is directly related to utilization of dental services. Dental treatment is the most sensitive of all the health services to variations in family income. Family income remains an important factor in determining whether individuals attend for dental care even when the financial barrier to receiving care is reduced. This indicates that socially determined patterns of behaviour associated with high incomes are often related to high – status occupations and good educational background, because these three factors are often positively associated with each other.

The 1971–73 National Health Survey data show an increase in annual dental visits per person from 1.0 at the $ 3,000 - $ 4999 income level to 2.0 at $ 15,000 and over. Analysis by Manning and Phelps of a data set shows that as the percentage of additional family income increases, there is a substantial percentage increase in the effective demand for dental care, although at a slightly lower rate. Thus, demand for dental care is "elastic" in its relationship to family income.

The correlation between income and utilization has been found to be more consistently positive when income is measured in terms of either being 'low' or 'high'. Newman and Anderson found that rise in income did not affect the mean number of visits for individuals in the 2–13 age group for income less than $ 5000, or in the 14–24 age group for incomes less than $ 3500. However, when income rose above these levels mean number of visits for these age groups rose correspondingly. A general pattern emerged for the 25–44 and 45–64 age groups with relatively low level of visits for family income of less than $ 5000, medium levels of visit for incomes form $ 5000 - $ 12,499 and the highest level of visits for incomes of $ 12,500 or more.

In a study by Salber et al; this same effect of income "threshold" was evident in that the proportion of blacks in one community seeing a dentist within the past year does not increase substantially for income categories less than $12,000 and year. However, the proportion of whites seeing a dentist within the past year was positively related for all incomes. Hoschtim et al, found no significant difference between the percent of blacks who had no dental checkups in more than two years whether classified as having adequate or inadequate incomes.

It is evident then that income, while having a strong positive relationship with utilization of dental services, does not fully explain difference in rates of utilization among segments of population. Therefore, one should guard against using only economic criteria in estimating the utilization rates when changes in the dental insurance status of the population are considered.

6. OCCUPATION:

Occupation is usually a product of education and a determinant of income.

Therefore, in looking at rates of utilization of dental services by occupation, the combined effect of these two factors becomes evident. While it is not feasible to rank all occupations according to status, they can be grouped with unskilled, semi-skilled and laborers as low status; skilled, clerical and sales as middle status; and executive and professional–managerial as high status.

A direct relationship exists between occupational status and frequency of dental visits. Persons in professional occupations visit their dentists more frequently than semi or non-skilled manual workers. Members of professional families are also more likely than manual workers to go for preventive visits. According to Anderson and Newman, high status occupations use dental services more than middle status and middle status occupations use dental services more than low status.

7. DENTAL INSURANCE:

People with dental insurance visit a dentist more often than people without insurance. The 1989 data showed that 71.4% of those with private dental insurance visited a dentist within the last year, compared with 50% of those without. These differences are to be expected but dental insurance can substantially reduce the financial burden of dental care. People with limited financial resources may give dental care a lower priority than other expenses that they perceive to be more urgent according to Milgrom P et al, 2004.[34] To explain the role of dental insurance, we have to look at who has it: professionals, white collar workers and the large labour unions who receive group dental care as a fringe benefit of employment. So again, there is likely to be a SES relationship, as well as some financial incentive for these groups.

8. SOCIOECONOMIC STATUS OR SOCIAL CLASS:

Socioeconomic status is the strongest determinant of dental care use and expenditure. The economic polarization within the society and lack of social security system makes the poor more vulnerable in terms of affordability and choice of health provider.[35] Poverty not only excludes people from the benefits of health care system but also restricts them from participating in decisions that affect their health, resulting in greater health inequalities. In most of the developing countries of south Asia region, it has been observed that magnitude of household out of pocket expenditure on health is at times as high as 80 percent of the total amount spent on health care per annum.[36] Not only the consultation fee or the expenditure incurred on medicines count but also the fare spent to reach the facility and hence the total amount spent for treatment turns out to be cumbersome. Consequently, household economics limit the choice and opportunity of health seeking.[37] In addition to being defined by income, education and occupation, socioeconomic status or social class involves beliefs, attitudes and behaviours that are inherent at each class level. There is a close relationship between social class and utilization of dental services, the higher the SES, the greater the use of dental services. As with gender differences, this relationship is found consistently in all industrialized countries, even in those where the cost barrier for dental care has been removed through public financing. The reasons for consistent relationship between SES and use of dental services are more complicated than they might appear. It is easy to say that lower SES people are less interested in oral health or less aware of the value of dental care. That often-heard assertion is rather over simplified.

Values and attitudes are naturally different, and many lesser educated people are from backgrounds in which dental care was virtually non-existent so there is none of the middle – class culture of which dental care is a part. More obviously, lower SES groups are less able to afford care when it does exist, and because there are fewer dentists in lower SES areas, care is usually less available. In Koos study, the value placed on healthy teeth was found to be positively correlated with social class. A study by the ADA went a step further to determine what attitudes toward dental care were predominant in each class. Basically, they found that the upper middle and lower middle class were concerned with the social value of good looking, clean teeth, while the upper lower and lower classes considered decay and less of teeth to be inevitable and, therefore, did not see the need for regular dental care. In an attempt to explain the relationship between SES and visit to the dentist, Kriesbery and Trieman, 1960 determined that early children training and the characteristics of the individual's dentist are more significant than information about teeth, beliefs about their care, and values about teeth.

Frazier et al, carried out a study which determined why dental care was not sought for children whose needs had been identified of the four SES groups in the study, there was no untreated need in the highest SE level, some in the second highest and lowest levels, and the greatest amount of untreated (decay) need in the second lowest level. The barriers to treatment named by the members of the lower three levels included cost, fear, family problems, lack of knowledge as to where to seek treatment, and distrust of the dentist. While it is evident then, that social class cannot be completely explained by income, education and occupation separately. The combination of these three variables could produce a strong factor in determining dental service utilization patterns.

9. ENVIORNMENTAL FACTORS:

The key categories of environmental factors that can influence individual behaviors and perceptions and, ultimately, have an impact on oral and general health status include political, social, and provider factors, as well as the predisposing, enabling and need variables. Oral and general health statuses are presented as the central component subject to the effects of individual behaviors and perceptions, which are influenced by the environment. The focal outcome measures of health status include actual, clinically measured, genetic, self-perceived health status and satisfaction indicators. Individual behaviors that contribute to oral health status are influenced by the environmental milieu, which consists of a dynamic inter play among cultural, community, interpersonal, media, policy/political, religion, socioeconomic and other variables. Many of the conditions are overlapping and may be secondary to underlying factors. For example, inter personal relationships, such as social support and marital status; have been found to be associated with health, morbidity, and mortality. This phenomenon is especially noted in minority populations. Religiosity has apparent beneficial effects on health in black populations which may be related to its role in providing social support or health education. Patient–provider relationships, including trust and racial pairing, also have been shown to affect health behaviors.

Health service utilization, a key behavior associated with oral health status, depends on the availability of and access to care. Suboptimal dental utilization may be a function of the health coverage accessible by the population. A higher proportion of minority than white individuals have never seen a dentist. Insurance is a recognized enabling variable, but the socioeconomic environment often determines the type or potential for having insurance. The type of health insurance (or lack of it) varies among different racial/ethnic groups. Black populations group are more likely than are whites to be covered by Medicaid and less likely to have private insurance, whereas Hispanics are least likely to have insurance coverage. Analyzing the role of this variable in influencing health behavior and health status requires care; in addition to availability of insurance, the individual must actively seek out and accept such assistance in access to care. Even for insured people, public and private insurers may alter health coverage and public policy may change, as was the case with the recent expansion of health care coverage for low income families enacted through the State Children's Health Insurance Program (SCHIP). California Health and Safety Code mandates improvements for low-income children with regard to access to dental care, including assistance with scheduling and transportation.

10. SOCIAL – PSYCHOLOGICAL FACTORS:

"Why do some people attend regularly for preventive and therapeutic care before symptoms appear while others attend only when they experience pain or discomfort?" Three inter related and interdependent social psychological explanations have been proposed to explain some of the variation in utilization. They are:

- Motivation
- Perception
- Learning.

A number of social – psychological explanations have been suggested to explain the prerequisites for utilizing health services and factors delaying action. Mechanic (1962) considered that a given illness has certain characteristics which will be perceived by a person and by associated significant others. The characteristics are

- Illness recognition
- Illness danger.

Illness recognition:

Includes the frequency with which the illness occurs in a population and the relative familiarity with the symptoms of the average member of the group.

Illness danger:

Includes knowledge of the relative predictability of the outcome of the illness and the amount of threat and loss likely to result from the illness.

When a symptom is both easily recognized and devoid of danger, it is a routine illness. Rarer symptoms which are difficult to identify and which are perceived to be more dangerous are likely to cause greater concern. Whether the individual finally presents fro treatment will depend on anxiety, fear of the dentist, financial and psychological factors.

The sequence of stages and decision making points in the illness behaviour and care seeking process are as follows[38];

a. The decision that something is wrong (symptom exercise and recognition).

b. The decision that one is sick and needs professional care. (Assumption of the sick role).

c. The decision to seek medical or dental care (Medical/dental care contact).

d. Decision to transfer control to the physician dentist. (Dependant patient role).

e. Decision to relinquish the patient role (Recovery and rehabilitation).

These theories of illness behaviour attempt to explain why individuals seek medical or dental care.

11. RACE AND ETHNICITY:

Race as a characteristic of utilization of dental services, has been measured in a number of studies and surveys by comparing the studies and surveys by comparing the user rates of whites with that of non whites. Whites use dental services more than non whites even when controlling for age and sex (Hochstin et al 1968).[39] In 1989, 59.3% of white Americans reported a visit within the last year as compared to 44.5% of African – Americans and 46.4% of Hispanic Americans. May be because of SES influences and the fact that these races have suffered historically from deliberate exclusion from many care facilities, and there are few dental providers from these groups. Some interesting variations in the use of dental services by race were found by Newman and Anderson (1972). Mean visits by non whites (2.1) were greater than mean visits by whites (1.9) when the education level of the head of the household was college and the occupation level was professional managerial (highest level). Okada and sparer (1976) found that the utilization rates were similar for blacks and whites according to data obtained in 1969–71. This was due to greater access to dental resources, greater availability of resources and broader Medicaid coverage. It appears that race per se dose not determine whether or not a person will seek dental care. Utilization data are not easy to interpret because race and ethnicity are inextricably related to wealth and poverty, education, cultural values and residential location.[40]

12. SOCIO-CULTURAL FACTORS:

Cultural beliefs and practices often lead to self-care, home remedies and consultation with traditional healers in rural communities. Advice of the elder women in the house is also very instrumental and cannot be ignored. These factors result in delay in treatment seeking and are more common amongst women, not only for their own health but especially for children's illnesses. Family size and parity, educational status and occupation of the head of the family are also associated with health seeking behaviour besides age, gender and marital status. However, cultural practices and beliefs have been prevalent regardless of age, socio-economic status of the family and level of education. An equitable use of health care amongst cultural and linguistic minority populations is one of the important goals within health care systems. Models for comprehensively understanding the equitable use of health care and for implementing effective interventions to reduce the disparities in health care are addressed. In particular, Jacobs and colleagues concluded that language barriers have negative consequences for linguistic minorities in accessing health care. Studies showed that the cultural and linguistic minority population has experienced more barriers in accessing health care due to socioeconomic disadvantages and limited English proficiency.

The disparities raised concerns with respect to health services utilisation amongst children living with families from non-English speaking background (NESB). In the United States (US), children from NESB were less likely than those from English speaking background (ESB) to have a regular source of health care; were almost two and half times less likely as ESB children to see a specialist physician; and were less likely to use after-hours emergency care. Similar evidence was also found in Canada and the United Kingdom (UK). The descriptive sociodemograhic approach to utilization of health services has severe limitations because although it describes certain broad trends, its explanatory power of the intervening variables and mechanisms is weak, greater attention should therefore be paid to the study of social and social – psychological factors. "The family, its relationship and friendship networks influences the manner in which individuals define and act upon symptoms or life crises". – McKinlay, 1972. Kriesbery and Treiman (1962) and Rayner (1970) showed the use of dental services is learned by example, particularly from mothers. Medical sociologists have suggested that the particular symptoms acted upon are defined by the culture, ethnic or reference group (Zole, 1966) and that the structure of the group and the health orientation and value system played an important role in defining utilization behaviours. [41-43]

13. ACCULTURATION:

Acculturation is defined as "those phenomena which result when groups of individuals having different cultures come into continuous first-hand contact, with subsequent changes in the original culture pattern of either group". This process does not occur at the same rate or to the same degree in all individuals.

During the last of the 20th century, the world we live in has become much smaller a place. As large numbers of people migrate to all corners of the globe, large and varied ethnic minorities have taken root where relatively homogenous populations once resided. Such a trend is seen not only in urban areas but also in rural places. In the 21st century, one can expect populations to become more and more culturally, racially and ethnically diverse. The diversity of the population as it relates to the myriad of ethnic groups represents a visible challenge to the health care providers. People with different ethnic and cultural backgrounds differ in their constructs of health and illness and how these constructs influence their perception of health.

When individuals migrate to other countries, they try to adjust to the new context. It is a highly complex process that includes socio-cultural adjustment as well as psychological adjustment. Socio-cultural adjustment involves language ability, cultural knowledge, and formation of social relationships while psychological adjustment involves change in beliefs, attitudes and preferences. The pattern of acculturation varies from one individual or other and also from one immigrant group to other.[44] The individual's strategy for acculturation may fall into three categories namely:-

a. **Assimilation**: Completely accepting and acquiring the new culture.

b. **Separation**: Maintenance of culture of origin through rejection or avoidance of new culture.

c. **Integration**: Embracing and valuing both the cultures. Usually, individuals who adopt this strategy experience lower acculturative stress than the above two strategies.

Acculturation makes a unique contribution to the oral health status above and beyond other socio-demographic variables. Higher levels of acculturation are associated with an increase in oral health knowledge. The impact of acculturation on oral health has been studied and overall positive results have been shown. Acculturation outcomes are further dictated by other social factors such as wealth, education, occupational skills, language ability, individual personality traits, structure and resources of the immigrants' families and communities, the extent to which the immigrants' presence is resented by the host community, the cultural distance between the new and old society, political and economic contexts of the new society and many more. Literature also suggests that not always acculturation leads to positive results. Acculturated Latinos living in United States were found to have undesirable dietary habits and engage more in substance abuse compared to their less acculturated counterparts.

The association between acculturation and oral diseases has been evaluated mostly with respect to caries and/or periodontal diseases. Overall, a positive impact of acculturation on oral health can be appreciated. Among Hispanics in the United States, the Hispanic Health and Nutrition Examination Survey, using a multidimensional acculturation scale, showed a reduced prevalence of gingivitis and periodontal pockets in highly acculturated adolescents and adults. In Hispanic adults with orofacial pain, those who were English-speaking or with high nativity suffered less from the pain and its complications. In another group of Hispanic adults, acculturation measured by English language proficiency indicated higher Oral Health Status Index, a score integrating the tooth and periodontium status. In Latino farm worker families, compared with foreign-born children, those local-born had a better oral health, as rated by their mothers. Among Hispanic preschool children, being born in the United States, speaking English, and mother's longer residence in the United States implied lower rate of early childhood caries. Also, it has been found that adults who immigrated to the United States at an older age had higher prevalence of caries and periodontal diseases and higher treatment needs. In a sample of adult Haitian immigrants living in New York City, higher acculturation, as defined by a multidimensional scale, was linked to lower rates of caries, periodontal attachment loss, and missing teeth.

A Canadian report showed that, the presence of calculus, gingivitis, caries and treatment needs among adolescent immigrants decreased with their length of residence among Portuguese-speaking immigrants. Parents who had immigrated in their 20s or at an older age were 2–4 times more likely to have a child with early childhood caries than those who immigrated at a younger age. In the United Kingdom, Asian women who spoke English were less likely to have a child with caries. In Sweden, adolescents who were second generation immigrants or who had arrived before one year of age had a caries prevalence similar to those of native adolescents, whereas those who arrived after seven years of age had a caries prevalence that was 2–3 times higher.

In Germany, a lower DMFT was found among local-born adolescent immigrants, as compared with their foreign-born counterpart. Compared with new arrivals, Pakistani immigrants who had lived in Norway for a longer period of time had better periodontal condition, indicated by the subgingival calculus and pocket depth. A study among Vietnamese in Australia showed that while behavioral acculturation reduced the caries rate in young adults not working outside home, the relationship between psychological acculturation and caries was non-linear, as laborers and students with a medium level of psychological acculturation had significantly higher DMFS scores than those with low or high acculturation.

A report among the elderly of multiple ethnic groups has demonstrated improvement in oral health-related quality of life with the length of residence in the United States. In the United Kingdom, favorable oral health knowledge of Japanese children was associated with being local-born. Also, satisfactory oral hygiene of Asian immigrant children was linked to mother's use of English language. In Australia, Vietnamese immigrants with medium level of acculturation had significantly lower oral health knowledge scores than those in the low and high acculturation categories.

Acculturation and Utilization of Dental Services:

Among Hispanics in the United States, data from Hispanic Health and Nutrition Examination Survey reveals better dental insurance coverage and more dental visits reported by adolescents and adults with higher acculturation, as measured by multidimensional scales. Such a trend was found in all three Hispanic groups namely Mexican-American, Cuban-American and Puerto Ricans. English-speaking Hispanic adults in Florida were more likely to have a dental home, as compared with non-English-speaking group. In a sample of Hispanics adults who were suffering from orofacial pain, those who were Spanish-speaking or more close to Hispanic culture were less likely to seek treatment and/or have a regular dentist. In Hispanic farm worker families, dental care was more received by children born in the United States. As to Hispanic preschoolers, dental visits were more common among those who were local born or English-speaking.

Studies among other ethnic minorities in the United States also demonstrated positive impacts of acculturation on utilization of dental care. The use of dental services increased with length of residence in the

United States among Chinese elderly immigrants and adults of Hispanic or Asian origins, but not among the Russian elderly. Higher level of English proficiency was associated with dental visit in Hispanic adults but not among Asians. In Canada, use of dental services increased with length of residence among the elderly population of Chinese origins. In the United Kingdom, local-born children of Japanese origin tended to visit dentists more often, compared with those born in Japan. Among Turkish immigrants in Germany, proficiency in German language indicated a tendency of using dental services. Similarly, among Pakistani immigrants in Norway, use of dental care increased as the duration their residence in the host country increased. Psychological acculturation facilitated dental visit of Vietnamese immigrants who were 35 years and above and who had spend 20% of their life in Australia.[44]

14. TRADITIONAL HEALERS:

A traditional healer is a person who has no formal medical training, but is recognized by the community in which he/she lives as being competent to provide health care by using plant, animal and mineral substances and certain other methods based on social, cultural and religious background as well as the knowledge, attitudes and beliefs that are prevalent in the community regarding physical, mental and social well-being and the causation of the disease and disability.

According to the World Heath Organization (WHO)[45], more than 80 per cent of population in developing countries relies on traditional medicine and indigenous knowledge to meet their health needs. This is due to the fact that traditional medicine is accessible, affordable, culturally and socially acceptable and most people prefer it to the 'exorbitantly priced' conventional Western medicine. With the legalization of traditional medicine as a complimentary health care service to primary health care in Cameroon, the role of the traditional healer was vital in the promotion of health especially in resource poor settings and rural areas where they may be the only source of health care.

Rural populations do not have access to the services of trained oral health personnel due to cost constraints and poor accessibility. Nearly twice as many people from poor households rely on traditional medicine as do people from rich households. Given shrinking health budgets, economic constraints and the diminishing capacity for oral health personnel to handle the burden of oral diseases, it would seem logical to develop and enhance co-operation and collaboration between the formal oral health services and Traditional Healers to bring available resources in the health sector to serve the population for better oral health. Traditional healers are considered to be effective agents of change as they command authority in their communities, function as psychologists, marriage and family counselors, physicians and legal and political advisors. They are also the legitimate interpreters of customary rules of conduct, morality and values. Traditional Healers provide client-centered, personalized health care that is culturally appropriate and tailored to meet the needs and expectations of the client paying special respect to social and spiritual matters.[46]

15. GENERAL HEALTH:

People who consider themselves in excellent health visit a dentist more often than those who see themselves as in good or only fair health. Among those who considered themselves to the in 'excellent' health, 61.9% reported a visit during 1989 compared with 51.5% who thought their health was 'good' and 39.8% who thought it was 'fair' or 'poor'. Distributions of a similar nature were found among those who had no restriction of activity compared with those who were limited to some degree. These findings are hardly unexpected because people whose mobility is restricted quite naturally would find getting to a dentist more difficult. Those in poor general health may be toot preoccupied, or too restricted generally, to face the dentist. These distributions also are likely to be related to age and perhaps to SES.

16. PUBLIC PRIVATE PARTNERSHIP:

Services provided by the public as well as the private sectors also determine the oral health seeking behaviour as well as utilization of dental services. In Finland, dental services were provided by a public and a private sector. Children, young adults and special needs groups were entitled to care and treatment from the public dental services (PDS). A major reform in 2001–2002 opened the PDS and extended subsidies for private dental services to all adults. It aimed to increase equity by improving adults' access to oral health care and reducing cost barriers. An evaluation was made of how the health political goals of the reform: integrating oral health care into general health care, improving adults' access to care and lowering cost barriers had been fulfilled during the study period. In 2000, when access to publicly subsidised dental services was restricted to those born in 1956 or later, every third adult used the PDS or subsidised private services. By 2004, when subsidies had been extended to the whole adult population, this increased to almost every second adult. The PDS reported having seen 118076 more adult patients in 2004 than in 2000. The private sector had the same number of patients but 542656 of them had not previously been entitled to partial reimbursement of fees. The use of both public and subsidised private services increased most in big cities and urban municipalities where access to the PDS had been poor and the number of private practitioners was high. The PDS employed more dentists (6.5%) and the number of private practitioners fell by 6.9%. The total dental care expenditure (PDS plus private) increased by 21% during the study period. Private patients who had previously not been entitled to reimbursements seemed to gain most from the reform. Combination of both private as well as public sector to promote oral health could reduce burden of oral diseases.

17. ORGANIZATIONAL FACTORS:

The way the health services are organized may be as important as the social psychological factors in determining patterns of utilization. Members of particular categories of society may not have the necessary expertise to cope with certain organizational structures and will therefore delay or avoid utilizing them according to Young and Willmott, 1959. Induced in some countries there is a wide gap between modern health care services and certain groups who have traditional beliefs according to Morley, 1974. Certain social class behaviours are patterned and systematically inter-related, attempts to change the behaviour rather creating organizational structures are often unsuccessful. Gillespie (1978) noted that in attempts to provide dental care, involving the community in the planning was the first and most important lesson. If change is to be effected, a mere increase in manpower is not enough. It is necessary to change the basis of the system and to radically change the system of delivery. More emphasis should be placed on organizational structures than on the personal pathologies of under-utilizers. Organizational structures which determine certain social classes should be modified.

18. OTHER FACTORS:

Inequality has been described as health differences which are avoidable, unnecessary unjust and unfair (whitehead, 1991). Inequalities have been observed between groups in a region and between geographic regions in the same country. In order to assess an inequality we must first judge the situation against the background or context of what is happening in society generally. Example: Dental decay declined in the UK in all social classes between 1983–1993, the gap in experience of dental decay has widened between 12–15 year olds from skilled households (who had improved most) and children from semi skilled and unskilled households (who had improved least). Evidence suggests that disadvantaged groups have poorer survival chances and a greater experience of illness during their life time compared to more favoured groups.

The determinants of health inequality: (White head, 1991).

a. Natural, genetic or biological variation.

b. Health damaging behaviour if freely chosen. Example: Participation in certain sports.

c. The transient health advantage when one group is the first to adopt a health promoting behaviour which then becomes wide spread.

d. Health damaging behaviour, where the choice of lifestyle is severely restricted. Example: Living in damp housing.

e. Exposure to unhealthy, stressful, living and working conditions.

f. Example: Miners and Chronic lung disease.

g. Inadequate access to essential health and other public services.

h. Example: Homeless people.

i. Natural selection or health related social mobility where there is a tendency for sick people to move down the social scale.

The first three determinants of inequality are neither unnecessary, unjust nor unfair. But the latter four clearly are and need to be addressed.

It is not feasible to devise strategies (which would include health promotion and the provision of health care services) to ensure everyone has the same standard of health and access to health care. Whitehead[47] suggests we should be looking to achieve a fair distribution throughout the country based on health care needs and case of access in each geographical area and the removal of barriers to access. To reduce health differentials, the principles of health promotion must be relied upon. By improving living conditions, providing supportive environments and cultivating greater participation of lay people in decision making, it is possible to considerably reduce the determinants of poor health. At the micro-level, inequality exists in terms of the outcomes of health care and the quality of care received. Middle class people usually get more consultation time with their doctor and are more likely to get referred for secondary care. They are also more likely to avail themselves of preventive services. The main barriers for dental services utilization include:

I. **The two main barriers:-**

Anxiety and Cost

Of the range of attitudes expressed in relation to dental services, two stand out as the most significant barriers to take up. One is an underlying apprehension or anxiety, the other is the cost of receiving dental treatment. The anxiety can be in general terms, or focusing on a particular aspect: for example fear of pain of a specific treatment or other potential for embarrassment or discomfort. Anxiety or fear of pain has been found to be a significant barrier to seeking preventive care by Kriesbery and Treiman, Freidson and Feldman, Antonovsky and Kats, Tash et al, and Kegeles. One cause of the fear of dental pain has been theoretically attributed to the various psychological associations of oral cavity with pain from infancy through adulthood: the mouth is the source of first pleasure through nursing, as well as the source of first pain with teething, and is later used for expressing affection as well as aggression. Consequently, since the mouth is so valuable there is a greater fear of the pain caused by dental treatment. Research does not fully support this theory, nor does it explain why some people are afraid to go to dentist and others are not. Metzner suggests that fear of pain may simply be based on past dental experiences.

Research on oral surgery patients by Debbs, et al, suggests that a patient's perceived sensitivity to pain and general fear about what will happen at the dental treatment are two of the major factors that can predict the amount of distress that will be experienced at a particular dental visit. Considering that lower socioeconomic level persons have more extractions than preventive treatment there could be more cause for these persons to fear visiting the dentist. According to the studies by Keiesberg and Treiman, fear and anxiety accounted for differences of preventive utilization at all income levels with no differences apparent between various socioeconomic levels. Kegeles et al found that anxiety and fear of pain were correlated negatively with dental visits. According to Lissau (1989) dental anxiety was a strong predictor among females, pain tolerance was a strong predictor among males.

II. **Economic barriers:**

Dental treatment is considered by many to be expensive and is openly acknowledged by some as a reason for rationale for postponing the dental visit especially after a lapse in attendance. From the economic literature, cost is seen as the major barrier to utilisation of treatment services. This barrier can exist in two primary ways. The actual price of the service is too high and the amount of disposable income available for buying the service is too low. Therefore, changes in either price or income will alter the cost barrier. Therefore, changes in either price or income will alter the cost barrier. Several economic analyses of price, income and demand data have appeared in the literature.

Anderson and Benham (1971), Feldstein (1973), Holtman and olsen (1972, 1976), Maurizi (1975) and Newhouse (1974) all report demand estimates. Lissau I et al, 1989 found perceived economic barriers correlated negatively with frequency of preventive dental visits. Holst found no increased use of services among young urban adult males with a high level of reimbursement and concluded that third party payment may be a necessary, but not a sufficient incentive for use of dental services. On the contrary, Craft and Croucher argued for removing the financial barriers in order to increase utilisation of dental services among young adults in the UK. Flemming Scheutz and Heidmann J [34] id not find any empirical evidence of any association between the participant's income and use of dental services. There was no difference in utilisation of dental services between those who had a private dental insurance and those who did not studies from the Nordic countries have concluded that public subsidy schemes have no or very little influence on the demand for dental care once copayments have been introduced. It is therefore unlikely that economic incentives alone would be effective in reaching the overall goal. Amit chattopadhyay found that dental insurance was an important determinant of oral care use.[13] Enhancing dental insurance significantly increased the dental visits.

III. **Perception of need (perceived need):**

These are the needs which people perceive as being important. They are subjective feelings of what people really want. An increased perception of need could be instrumental in establishing a regular pattern of attendance. With a low perception of need, the other barriers remain significant. In a study by Hester V et al lack of perceived need was a barrier to care in 86% of elderly subjects. This is because among the frail and functionally dependent elderly people dental handicap is realized as a lower priority ailment than others. Scheectz F and Heidmann J (2001) found that perceived poor condition of the teeth was a good predictor of being a regular user. But Kari Stoirhang found that those with the most negative perception of their own dental health were the most irregular attenders.

The decision to seek certain kinds of health care is determined by the relative significance the individual attaches to the symptoms of illness and his belief regarding the most appropriate response to these symptoms. Newman and Anderson reported that the major reason for dental visits among the general population in the US is related to the individual perception that a dental problem does infact exist. Other authors have stated that perceived need for care is one of the key determinants of both self-care and in seeking provider based services.

Perceived need, as apposed to objectively assessed need, has emerged in many studies as one of the most accurate predictors of both medical and dental services use. Branch et al (1986) operationalised perceived need as the individual's self report of health status and limitations in activities of daily living. Erashwrick et al. (1982) found the perceived need number of dental problems to be the best predictor of both recency and number of dental visits among their sample of persons over 62. A survey of 1573 elderly in Finland by Tuominen and Paunio, 1986 revealed that perceived need, as operationalised by tooth aches and oral discomfort, was a better predictor of utilisation than income or dentist: patient ratio in the region. Knazan (1986) found that 74% of those who had not seen a dentist in more than 5 years gave as a reason that they felt no need. Similar results were found by Konigsberg (1983). A study done by Eddie in Scotland suggests that having a perceived need for dental care is not sufficient to evoke a dental visit and many people visit a dentist without perceiving any specific treatment need e.g. for a check up or for preventive services. People's past dental services utilisation behaviour is probably one of the most important predictors of their future utilisation behaviours. It seems that once the subjects established a certain pattern of dental visit behaviour, they would maintain that pattern irrespective of their oral health status and perceived need for treatments.

People who underestimate their own dental health or dental care needs relative to clinical assessments will use fewer services. Reisine and Bailit found that people tend to rate their oral health more favorably than clinical indications would warrant. People tend to overestimate their dental health and underestimate their need for care. Such misperceptions stand in the way of active care seeking behaviour.

IV. **Access barriers:**

Access to dental care has been correlated with utilisation of dental services in many studies. Although finding a dentist may not be a problem for many people, other aspects of access could present barriers. The journey to reach the dentist, in terms of time and cost, was a factor discussed in the rural field work area, and in general, travel costs were mentioned as a consideration in the selection of a dentist nearby.

More significant for some working people was an apparent difficulty in disrupting one's routine in order to find the time to a) organise and b) attend a dental appointment.

When combined with a low perception of the need for dental visits, this problem assumed greater emphasis or if a high degree of apprehension and anxiety was already a problem, the waiting time between making the appointment and walking into the surgery could give rise to; as much if not more apprehension as the receipt of the treatment itself. Access to dental care was correlated with utilisation of preventive dental services by Kegeles in a study where he found that "36% of the people who lived more than 10 miles from the city where the clinic was located made preventive dental visits as compared with 59% of those who lived within ten miles of the clinic city".

Access to dental care is not limited to a measure of the distance from the patient to the dentist, but includes the time, costs of waiting time for an appointment, the availability of a dentist, who will agree to special financial arrangements for certain patients, and the convenience of keeping an appointment. The time barrier includes the value of the patient's travel time, waiting time, and treatment time. Consequently; for anyone who will lose income from taking work time off to obtain barrier, whether they be Rs. 10/hours for an hourly wage earner or Rs. 100/hour for an executive.

The convenience of the dental appointment is closely related to the socioeconomic level. More likely than not, the lower social level person is paid by hourly wages and does not have great flexibility in setting work hours whereas the higher level professional is usually paid by salary and has more freedom to set his own work time. Consequently, it is more costly for the lower socioeconomic level person to take time off for a dental appointment, as well as being more complicated since he must request leave and may experience greater transportation problems.

According to Helen Finch, an apparent difficulty in disrupting one's routine in order to find time to organise and attend a dental appointment is a significant barrier for some working people. Similar reason was cited as a barrier to utilisation of dental care in studies by Lahti SM et. al (1999).

V. **The image of dentists:**

According to Finch et al, dentists were regarded by those interviewed as ordinary people doing their job: individual approaches might vary with personality just as they might in any other profession. Yet as a profession it was felt that they suffered from a problem of association. When thinking of dentists, people thought of the potential for hurt/pain/discomfort that several associated with dental treatment, even if they had not actually experienced it. Two further aspects emerged as being strongly associated with the image of dentists; one was that dentists were considered impersonal in their approach to their patients, preoccupied with the physical or mechanical techniques of dentistry. 'They see you as a mouth' was a common way of expressing this, or a view of the dentist 'as a car mechanic'. This was reinforced by the additional view that dentists were highly paid, concerned with money, and supposedly therefore wanting to treat patients as much and/or as fast as possible in order to obtain their high level of income. This 'conveyor belt' image added to the impersonal image. Lack of acceptability of dentists and dental treatment was found by Frazier et al to be a substantial barrier preventing some people from seeking dental care. Cases are cited where people did not intend to go to the dentist until their teeth hurt because they did not believe in the need for dental treatment or had no confidence in dentists.

According to Freidson and Feldman those groups in the population who don't visit their dentist regularly as extensively as others also don't believe as extensively in the value of regular visits. These attitudes imply that there is a segment of the population which does not accept dental treatment as a viable alternative to decay and loss of teeth. According to studies by Kiyak and Miller, 1982[48]; dental attitude is one the most powerful predictors of dental care utilisation. According to Fishbein and Ajzen's (1972) summation model of attitudes, the importance attributed to oral health has emerged as a better discriminator than the generalised oral health beliefs held by individuals. According to Kiyak HA (1989)[48], patient and family attitudes described as lack of interest were perceived to be the second most important barrier to utilisation of dental services (50–70%).

Beliefs about illness and disease: Another way of looking at the discrepancy between need and demand is to consider people's norms and beliefs.

- An individual is unlikely to seek help if he or she does not consider symptoms to be important.

- Some potentially serious dental problems do not cause severe pain, being rather insidious in nature.

- Periodontal disease can develop gradually, not giving symptoms until the teeth become loose.

- An unattended periapical abscess can develop; into a chronic infection and ultimately a cyst which could compromise other teeth and bony support.

- If an individual is not aware of these facts and the role of screening, preventive action will not be taken. Even if pain is experienced it will be tolerated. Many people accommodate to low grade dental pain or a bad taste in the mouth and an impaired appearance.

SUMMARY & TAKE AWAY NOTES

Health in itself has got a great value. Social disparities in health and oral health outcomes as measured by education, occupation, income and household assets or by indices derived by combining indicators constitute one of the main challenges for Public health as well as dental public health. Health seeking behaviour is one of the major component of health. In recent years, epidemiologists and social scientists have devoted increasing attention to studying health-seeking behavior. Studies related to health seeking behaviour are based upon various models which are very often utilized and incorporated in several studies. None of the models are comprehensive by nature, so a combination of many or few models could be utilized to understand health seeking behaviour and its relationship or effect on health and in turn oral health.

Lower socio-economic and ethnic minority groups are less likely to utilize health services and might have poor oral health seeking behaviour. There is increasing demand for care among people of all age groups and there is limited availability of resources. Increased emphasis on oral health promotion and disease prevention appears to be the only feasible response. Health promotion is the ability of individuals to have control over the determinants of their health. Health promotion is the best way to tackle poor oral health seeking behaviour. Several other strategies could be implemented at individual level as well as community level to improve the health of those who have a poor oral health seeking behaviour.

Summary & Take Away Notes

Take Away Notes:

1. Various factors are implicated in determining the health and in turn health seeking behaviour of individuals. A majority of health problems are related to behavior of individuals which could determine health/oral health seeking behavior.

2. Utilization of dental services, availability of dental services, and accessibility to oral health as well as affordability determines the oral health seeking behaviour of individuals.

3. Various psychosocial determinants which influence health seeking behavior of individuals are socioeconomic status, education, occupation, income, religion, political factors, cultural factors including acculturation, custom, attitude, lifestyle and organizational factors.

4. Understanding oral health/health seeking behaviour of individuals is very complex and several authors tried to explain it through various models. One of the oldest models to explain health seeking behaviour includes health belief model followed by other models such as theory of planned behaviour, theory of reasoned action, health care utilization model and oral health care utilization model by Anderson and Newmann. By utilizing these models several studies are conducted to know about the relationship between health seeking behaviour with several parameters such as tooth brushing frequency, flossing, dental caries, periodontal disease and health care utilization. This valuable information obtained from these studies can be utilized to improve the oral health at individual and community level.

5. Several preventive and curative strategies implemented at community level or at individual level to maintain health could be useful only when individuals pay more attention towards their oral health and have a good oral health seeking behaviour.

REFERENCES

1. Ekkekakis P, Petruzzello SJ. Acute aerobic exercise and affect: current status, problems and prospects regarding dose-response. Sports Med. 1999 Nov;28(5):337–74. Review.

2. Nassani MZ, Kay EJ. Tooth loss—an assessment of dental health state utility values. Community Dent Oral Epidemiol. 2011 Feb;39(1):53–60.

3. Goldman N, Heuveline P. Health-seeking behaviour for child illness inGuatemala. Trop Med Int Health. 2000 Feb;5(2):145–55.

4. Baker SR. Applying Andersen's behavioural model to oral health: what are the contextual factors shaping perceived oral health outcomes? Community Dent Oral Epidemiol. 2009 Dec;37(6):485–94.

5. Roberts-Thomson KF, Stewart J, Giang Do L. A longitudinal study of the relative importance of factors related to use of dental services among young adults. Community Dent Oral Epidemiol. 2011 Jun;39(3):268–75.

6. Sheeran P and Abraham C. The Health Belief Model, in Predicting Health Behaviour (Conner, M. & Norman, P. eds.). 1995, Buckingham: Open University Press.

7. Conner M and Sparks P. The Theory of Planned Behaviour and Health Behaviours, in Predicting Health Behaviour (Conner, M. & Norman, P. eds.). 1995, Buckingham: Open University Press.

References

8. Andersen R and Neuman JF. Societal and individual determinants of medical care utilization in the United States. Milbank Memorial Fund Quaterly/Health and Society, 1975: 51:95–124.

9. Kroeger A. Anthropological and socio-medical health care research in developing countries. Social Science & Medicine1983, 17:147–161.

10. Good CM. Etnomedical Systems in Africa. 1987 New York: The Guilford Press.

11. Andersen RM: Revisiting the behavioral model and access to medical care: does it matter? J Health Soc Behav 1995, 36:1–10.

12. K.A. Atchison, L.F. Dubin/Dent Clin N Am 47 (2003) 21–39.

13. Brennan DS, Luzzi L, Roberts-Thomson KF. Dental service patterns among private and public adult patients in Australia. BMC Health Serv Res. 2008 Jan 3;8:1.

14. Cohen LK: Converting unmet need for care to effective demand. Int Dent J 1987; 37: 114 – 6.

15. Finch H, Keegan J, Ward K, SanyalSen B: Barriers to the Receipt of Dental Care: a qualitative study. London: Social and Community Planning Research; 1988.

16. Nash Ojanuga D and Gilbert C. Women's access to health care in developing countries. Social Science & Medicine, 1992; 35(4):613–617.

17. U.S. Department of Health and Human Services. *Oral Health in America: A Report of the Surgeon General.* Rockville, MD: U.S. Department of Health and Human Services, National Institute of Dental and Craniofacial Research, National Institutes of Health, 2000:2–3. (http://www.nidcr.nih.gov/)

References

18. U.S. Department of Health and Human Services. *Healthy People 2010.* 2nd ed. 2 vols. Washington, DC: U.S. Government Printing Office, November 2000. (http://www.healthypeople.gov/)

19. Interventions to Prevent Dental Caries, Oral and Pharyngeal Cancers, and Sports-related Craniofacial In- juries: Systematic Reviews of Evidence, Recommendations from the U.S. Task Force on Community Preventive Services, and Expert Commentary. *Am J Prev Med* 2002; 1–84; 23(1S).

20. U.S. Preventive Services Task Force. *Guide to Clinical Preventive Services*, 2nd Edition, Williams and Wilkins, Baltimore. 1996; 953p.

21. Brown LJ, Lazar V. Minority dentists: why do we need them? Closing the gap. Washington Office of Minority Health, U.S. Department of public health.

22. Dounglass CW and Cole KO Utilization of dental services in the United States. Journal of Dental Education 1979, 43(4): 223–35.

23. Varenne B, Petersen PE, Fournet F, Msellati P, Gary J, Ouattara S, Harang M, Salem G. Illness-related behaviour and utilization of oral health services among adult city-dwellers in Burkina Faso: evidence from a household survey. BMC Health Serv Res. 2006 Dec 27;6:164.

24. Virtanen JI, Berntsson LT, Lahelma E, et al. Children's use of GP services in the five Nordic countries. J Epidemiol Community Health 2006;60:162–7.

25. Finch H. Barriers to the receipt of dental care. Br dent J 1988: 195–196.

■ References ■

26. Borreani E, Wright D, Scambler S, Gallagher JE. Minimising barriers to dental care in older people. BMC Oral Health. 2008 Mar 26;8:7.

27. Al-Shammari KF, Al-Ansari JM, Al-Khabbaz AK, Honkala S. Barriers to seeking preventive dental care by Kuwaiti adults. Med PrincPract. 2007;16(6):413–9.

28. Skaret E, Raadal M, Kvale G, Berg E. Gender-based differences in factors related to non-utilization of dental care in young Norwegians. A longitudinal study. Eur J Oral Sci. 2003 Oct;111(5):377–82.

29. Nyyssönen V: Use of oral health services and adult oral health in Finland. Proc Finn Dent Soc 1992; 88:33–38.

30. Kelly M, Steele J, Nuttall N, Bradnock G, Morris J, Nu nn J, Pine C, Pitts N, Treasure E, White D: Adult Dental Health Survey: Oral Health in the United Kingdom 1998. London, The Stationery Office, 2000.

31. Sohn W, Ismail AI: Regular dental visits and dental anxiety in an adult dentate population. J Am Dent Assoc 2005;136:58–66.

32. Sanders AE, Spencer AJ, Slade GD. Evaluating the role of dental behaviour in oral health inequalities. Community Dent Oral Epidemiol. 2006 Feb;34(1):71–9.

33. Kikwilu EN, Masalu JR, Kahabuka FK, Senkoro AR. Prevalence of oral pain and barriers to use of emergency oral care facilities among adult Tanzanians. BMC Oral Health. 2008 Sep 29;8:28.

34. Patrick DL, Lee RS, Nucci M, Grembowski D, Jolles CZ, Milgrom P. Reducing oral health disparities: a focus on social and cultural determinants. BMC Oral Health. 2006 Jun 15;6 Suppl 1:S4.

35. Cost recovery in Ghana: are there any changes in health care seeking behaviour? Health Policy Plan 1998; 13: 181– 8.

• References •

36. Ha NT, Berman P, Larsen U. Household utilization and expenditure on private and public health services in Vietnam. Health Policy Plan 2002; 17: 61–70.

37. Quiñonez C, Grootendorst P. Equity in dental care among Canadian households. Int J Equity Health. 2011 Apr 16;10(1):14.

38. Garcha V, Shetiya SH, Kakodkar P. Barriers to oral health care amongst different social classes in India.Community Dent Health. 2010 Sep;27(3):158–62.

39. Dolan TA, Atchison KA. Implications of access, utilization and need for oral health care by the non-institutionalized and institutionalized elderly on the dental delivery system. J Dent Educ. 1993 Dec;57(12):876–87. Review.

40. Hunte P, Sultana F. Health seeking behavior and the meaning of medications in Balochistan, Pakistan. Soc Sci Med 1992; 34: 1385–1397.

41. Geissler PW et al. Children and medicines: self treatment of common illnesses among Luo schoolchildren in western Kenya. Soc Sci Med 2000; 50: 1771–83.

42. Perez-Cuevas R et al. Mother's health seeking behavior in acute diarrhea in Tlaxcala, Mexico. J Diarrhoeal Dis Res 1996; 14:260–8.

43. Cruz GD, Shore R, Le Geros RZ, Tavares M. Effect of acculturation on objective measures of oral health in Haitian immigrants in New York City. J Dent Res. 2004 Feb;83(2):180–4.

44. Kakatkar G, Bhat N, Nagarajappa R, Prasad V, Sharda A, Asawa K, Agrawal A. Barriers to the utilization of dental services in udaipur, India. J Dent (Tehran). 2011 Spring;8(2):81–9. Epub 2011 Jun 30.

References

45. Saddki N, Yusoff A, Hwang YL. Factors associated with dental visit and barriers to utilisation of oral health care services in a sample of antenatal mothers in Hospital Universiti Sains Malaysia. BMC Public Health. 2010 Feb 22;10:8.

46. Knowledge and practice of traditional healers in oral health in the Bui Division, Cameroon. J Ethnobiol Ethnomed 2011, 7:6. http://www.ethnobiomed.com/content/7/1/6.

47. Stuyft PV, Sorenson SC, Delgado E, Bocaletti E. Health seeking behavior for child illness in rural Guatemala. Trop Med Int Health 1996; 1: 161–70.

48. Kiyak HA. Reducing barriers to older persons' use of dental services. Int Dent J. 1989 Jun;39(2):95–102. Review.

www.ingramcontent.com/pod-product-compliance
Lightning Source LLC
Chambersburg PA
CBHW030903180526
45163CB00004B/1680